About the Authors

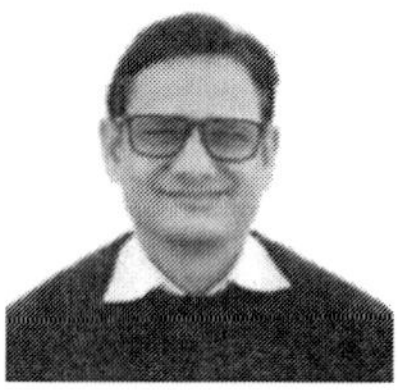

Dr. Kamalesh Kumar Meena is presently working as an Assistant Professor & In-charge Head in the Department of Dairy and Food Microbiology, College of Dairy and Food Technology, MPUAT, Udaipur, India. He has obtained his B.Tech. degree in Dairy Technology from CDFT, Udaipur (Raj.), M. Tech. degree in Dairy Microbiology from the National Dairy Research Institute, Karnal (Haryana), and Ph.D. from the National Institute of Food Technology and Entrepreneurship Management, Kundli (Haryana). **Dr. Meena** has 11 years' experience and fulfilled the mandate of teaching, research and extension. He is actively working in the area of probiotics, lactic acid bacteria, new product development, fermented foods and food safety. He has authored more than 40 papers in reputed journals, published 6 books, 22 practical manuals, and 11 book chapters/technical/popular articles. He was awarded best teacher award by MPUAT, Udaipur and ATDS, Ghaziabad. He served as a **Senior Executive** in the Quality Assurance Department of the Gujarat Cooperative Milk Marketing Federation Ltd. (Well-known as "AMUL"), Anand (Gujarat) for five years. He has an **Internal Auditor Certificate** from **Den Net Vertis (DNV), Germany** to conduct internal quality audits in the dairy and food industry. He was actively involved in manpower training given to food industry personnel for food safety and management. He has also handled various additional administrative responsibilities (Assistant Dean of Student Welfare, Hostel Warden, Head of Department, Programme Officer (NSS), In-charge Games & Sports, and ICAR, Nodal Officer for college) in addition to his routine duties of teaching and research.

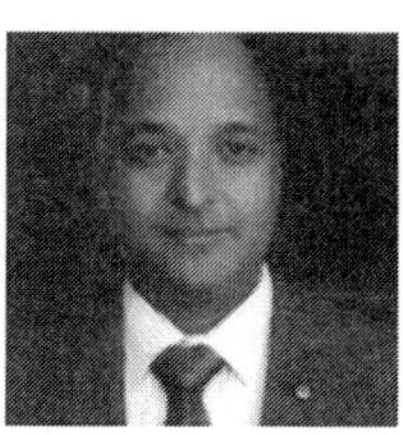

Dr. Lokesh Gupta, Professor, is presently working as Dean, College of Dairy and Food Technology, Maharana Pratap University of Agriculture and Technology, Udaipur. Dr. Gupta completed his Masters in 2000 with Gold Medal and doctorate degree in Animal Production in 2003. Dr. Gupta has 20 years experience and fulfilled the mandate of teaching, research and extension. His area of interest is organic poultry farming, feeding of area specific mineral mixture and production and utilization of azolla in the diets of dairy animals and poultry. He is a recipient

Fundamentals of Microbiology

NIPA® GENX ELECTRONIC RESOURCES & SOLUTIONS P. LTD.
New Delhi-110 034

of 17 awards including Bharatiya Govansha Sambardhan Pratishthan, Award in Animal Energy by Indian Society of Agricultural Engineering (ISAE), New Delhi; Fellow Award by Animal Nutrition Association, IVRI, Izatnagar, Fellow Award (SEE) by Society of Extension Education, Agra.

Best Paper Award by International Congress for Animal Reproduction, Vancouver (Canada); Best Teacher Award by MPUAT, Udaipur and many more by different National level organizations. He has published more than 76 research papers, 16 books, manuals, book chapters, articles and documentaries. He is associated with 24 externally funded projects. Dr. Gupta has organized many programmes for skill and entrepreneurship development in Agriculture including workshops/seminars/summer/ winter schools for the students, rural youths and faculties of State Agricultural Universities and Research Institutes of the country. He has visited Vietnam, Canada, Australia and Philippines for presentation of research papers and as a part of delegation for exploring the opportunities of research and teaching exchange programme.

Dr. Gupta has developed 66 technologies on different innovative/niche areas of Animal Production viz., area specific mineral mixture, draught animal power camel nutrition, azolla production and utilization, organic poultry farming, herbal feed supplementation, ethno-veterinary remedies etc which are also included in the Package of Practice (PoP) of Department of Agriculture Government of Rajasthan. He generated Rs. 402.00 lakh as revenue for the university from production and supply of poultry germplasm, mineral mixture Vermicompost, dairy produce etc. during 2018-2023.

Dr. Lokesh Gupta has identified and registered three new goat breeds as Sojat Goat, Karauli Goat and Gujari Goat in the year 2022. He developed 11 infrastructures including Mineral Mixture Production Unit, Azolla Production Unit, Organic Poultry Production Unit, Animal Nutrition Laboratories Demonstration and Meat Processing Unit, Poultry Brooder House, Goat Rearing Unit, Automatic Poultry Housing Unit, Skill Development Centre, Smart Classrooms and Conference Hall equipped with all IT gadgets for the university.

Fundamentals of Microbiology

Kamalesh Kumar Meena
Assistant Professor & In-charge Head
Department of Dairy and Food Microbiology
College of Dairy and Food Technology
Maharana Pratap University of Agriculture and Technology
Udaipur, Rajasthan

Lokesh Gupta
Professor & Dean
College of Dairy and Food Technology
Maharana Pratap University of Agriculture and Technology
Udaipur, Rajasthan

nipa®

NIPA® GENX ELECTRONIC RESOURCES & SOLUTIONS P. LTD.
New Delhi-110 034

NIPA® GENX ELECTRONIC RESOURCES & SOLUTIONS P. LTD.

101,103, Vikas Surya Plaza, CU Block
L.S.C. Market, Pitam Pura, New Delhi-110 034
Ph : +91-11-43860225, Mob.: +91 9717133558, 9540816132
E-mail: newindiapublishingagency@gmail.com
Website: www.nipaersources.com

Print ISBN: 978-93-58872-20-0
ebook ISBN: 978-93-58875-80-5

Composed and Designed by NIPA®.

Preface

Microbiology is the scientific discipline that focuses on the study of microorganisms, which are organisms too small to be seen with the naked eye. These microorganisms include bacteria, viruses, fungi, algae, and protozoa, each of which plays a unique role in ecosystems and human life. Despite their small size, microorganisms have an immense impact on health, the environment, and industrial processes. Microbiology encompasses various subfields, including microbiological genetics, which studies the heredity of microorganisms, and microbial physiology, which focuses on how microbes grow and interact with their environments. The discipline has direct applications in medicine, where microbiologists work to identify pathogens, develop vaccines, and combat antibiotic resistance. It also plays a key role in biotechnology, food science, agriculture, and environmental science, with microorganisms being used in the production of antibiotics, biofuels, and in waste management. In essence, microbiology is foundational to understanding life on Earth and addressing global challenges.

This book aims to introduce students to the various aspects of life in the microbial world. While microbiology covers a broad range of organisms, including bacteria, fungi, viruses, algae, and protozoa, its primary focus here is on the core techniques essential to the field. These foundational methods are key in preparing students to tackle the more advanced task of identifying pathogenic microorganisms in food, clinical and environmental samples. Each experiment begins with a brief theoretical overview, which not only explains the scientific principles behind the procedure but also helps bridge the gap between theory and practice. Safety protocols, critical for anyone working in microbiology, are also emphasized throughout.

Designed for students studying general microbiology—especially those involved in dairy and food product analysis—this laboratory book offers essential knowledge of microbiological techniques and experiments. Topics include the use of basic microbiological equipment, different types of microscopes, staining techniques, microbial size measurements, as well as methods for preparing broths and media. It also covers various plating techniques, serial dilution, and microbiological analysis of environmental samples such as soil, water, and air.

Authors

Contents

General Guidelines for the Microbiological Laboratory

Microbiologists are constantly at risk of exposure to hazardous microorganisms that can cause diseases. These microorganisms may enter the body through inhalation, ingestion, cuts, abrasions, or the eyes. Therefore, handling cultures, slides, and live microorganisms requires utmost care. To ensure safety in the laboratory, several precautions must be followed:

1. Maintain cleanliness in microbiological labs at all times, taking extra care to prevent contamination from the air, equipment, personnel, or the environment.
2. Always wear a clean white lab coat or apron while working. After handling infectious microorganisms, the lab coat should be autoclaved.
3. No eating, drinking, or smoking is allowed in the laboratory.
4. Personal hygiene is essential in microbiological labs.
5. Wash hands with soap and water or a mild disinfectant solution (e.g., hypochlorite solution containing 50-100 ppm chlorine or 1-2% lysol solution) before starting work.
6. Disinfect the work surface by wiping down the lab bench with a disinfectant solution, such as 5% phenol or hypochlorite solution containing 200-300 ppm chlorine, both before and after work.
7. Keep the work area neat and organized at all times.
8. Use self-adhesive labels instead of moistening labels with your tongue.
9. Sterilize inoculating loops and needles by heating them in a Bunsen burner flame until red hot before and after use.
10. Always store test tubes in test tube racks, not on the bench.
11. Treat all bacterial cultures as infectious. In case of breakage, immediately disinfect the area and transfer the materials to a separate container with a strong disinfectant.
12. Handle sporulating fungal cultures with care as they can cause respiratory infections or allergic reactions.

13. When working with food samples on nutrient agar, handle with caution as pathogenic microbes may grow.
14. Do not pipette by mouth. Use rubber bulbs, teats, or automatic pipettes.
15. Place all used pipettes in a disinfectant solution in a designated pipette jar. Dispose of all solid waste in proper containers—never in the sink or on the work surface.
16. Handle glassware and equipment carefully to avoid breakage. Report any damage immediately.
17. Report accidents such as spilled cultures, cuts, or ingestion of chemicals to the instructor.
18. Be aware of the location of first aid kits, irrigation bottles, and fire extinguishers. A list of hazards from chemicals and microorganisms should be available in the lab.
19. Clean the work area thoroughly with a suitable disinfectant after completing tasks.
20. Wash hands thoroughly before leaving the laboratory.

Keep a detailed record of experimental data and results in your laboratory notebook, and follow the prescribed format when submitting your report to the instructor.

1

Operating and Functional Principles of Basic Microbiology Laboratory Equipment

Introduction

In microbiological laboratories, various specialized equipment and apparatus are essential for conducting experiments and ensuring accurate results. Students of microbiology should familiarize themselves with the key features, operation, precautions, and maintenance of these instruments. Below is a description of some commonly used equipment in microbiological labs:

1. **Hot Air Oven:** This instrument is used for sterilizing heat-resistant materials like glassware, scalpels, syringes, and throat swabs. Sterilization is achieved through dry heat, typically at 160°C for 1-2 hours, which kills microorganisms by denaturing proteins, oxidizing cell components, and causing the toxic effects of elevated temperatures. The oven consists of a rectangular chamber with double walls—an outer layer made of mild steel or wood and an inner layer of stainless steel or aluminum. The space between the walls is insulated with materials like asbestos glass wool. Air is heated electrically, and the temperature is regulated by a thermocouple, ensuring uniform distribution with the help of fans. Proper ventilation and not overloading the oven are crucial for effective sterilization.
2. **Autoclave:** The autoclave is used for sterilizing surgical tools and bacteriological media using moist heat at temperatures above 100°C (usually 121°C for 15-20 minutes). Moist heat is more effective than dry heat because it penetrates better and has a higher lethal action on microorganisms. The autoclave operates under high steam pressure in a large cylindrical vessel made of durable metals like gunmetal or bronze. It includes a pressure gauge, thermometer, and steam valve to control steam release. A removable rack inside holds materials to be sterilized, which are exposed to 15 psi steam pressure for thorough sterilization.

Autoclaves are used for sterilizing liquid media, discarded cultures, contaminated glassware, and various other materials.

3. **Arnold Steam Sterilizer:** The Arnold steam sterilizer is used for fractional sterilization (also known as Tyndallisation), which is suitable for sterilizing heat-sensitive media such as gelatin, milk, and carbohydrate-based media. This method involves exposing media to free-flowing steam at 100°C for 30 minutes on three consecutive days, with an incubation period between exposures. This process effectively kills heat-resistant spores that germinate during incubation. The Arnold sterilizer is similar to an autoclave but operates at lower pressure and is constructed with mild steel or copper walls.
4. **Inspissator:** An inspissator is designed for sterilization at temperatures below 100°C, specifically for media containing sensitive substances like blood serum. It consists of a double-jacketed metallic water bath that is insulated and heated by an immersion heater. The temperature is controlled by a thermostat, and media tubes are sterilized by heating the water to 60-75°C for 6-8 hours.
5. **Incubator:** The incubator is a controlled environment chamber used for growing bacterial cultures. It maintains constant temperature and humidity, and often includes racks or shelves for holding culture tubes and Petri dishes. Heating is provided by electric coils or strip heaters, and the temperature is regulated by a thermostat. A BOD incubator is used to maintain temperatures below room temperature for specific biological applications.
6. **Water Bath:** A water bath is used to heat substances, such as milk or chemicals, in a controlled and uniform manner. The bath consists of double-walled copper or stainless steel, well-insulated, and electrically heated with thermostatic control. It is particularly useful for conducting tests like Methylene Blue or Resazurin tests, where consistent heating at a specific temperature is required.
7. **Refrigerator**: A refrigerator is used for storing cultures, milk samples, and certain chemicals at temperatures below 5°C. It consists of a finely finished enameled cabinet, an enclosed cooling coil system, and a compressing unit that uses ammonia or Freon. The refrigerator is equipped with compartments for different materials, as well as deep fridge chambers for storage. Temperature is controlled automatically through a thermostat.
8. **Laminar Air Flow Chambers**: Laminar air flow chambers are used for tasks like sub-culturing and plating. In these chambers, air passes

through high-efficiency particulate air (HEPA) filters made of cellulose acetate plates around aluminum foil, capable of removing particles as small as 0.3μm. The filtered air flows in parallel lines with consistent velocity throughout the enclosure. The chamber also includes a UV light for sterilization.

9. **Electronic Colony Counter**: An electronic colony counter is used to count bacterial colonies that form on solid media in a Petri dish after incubation. The device consists of a magnifying lens mounted on a stand to assist in the counting process.
10. **Lovibond pH Comparator**: The Lovibond pH comparator measures the hydrogen ion concentration (pH) of bacteriological media and other liquids by adding an indicator and comparing the resulting color with calibrated color discs for various pH values. It includes a vertical stand, a glazed glass plate for illuminating test tubes, and a slit for reading the pH disc, which is a series of small colored discs corresponding to specific pH ranges.
11. **Resazurin Comparator**: The resazurin comparator is used to measure the color change or reduction stage of resazurin in milk using a standard color disc. Its design is similar to the pH comparator but modified for resazurin tests. The disc is placed on a rectangular frame, with side openings for viewing the milk tubes placed beneath it, allowing the color to be compared with the standard disc.
12. **Colorimeter**: A colorimeter measures the concentration of biochemical compounds by analyzing how certain wavelengths of white light are absorbed by a colored solution. It works by passing light from a tungsten lamp through a slit, a condenser lens, and into a solution contained in a cuvette. The light passing through the solution is filtered to allow only wavelengths complementary to the color of the solution. The amount of absorbed light is then measured by a photocell, which provides a reading of absorbance or percent transmission.
13. **pH Meter**: A pH meter measures the pH of a solution using a glass electrode sensitive to hydrogen ions. The glass electrode contains a hydrogen chloride solution and is connected to a platinum wire via a silver-silver chloride electrode. A potential is generated across the glass, dependent on the pH of the solution. A reference electrode completes the circuit. Some pH meters combine both electrodes in a single unit. This meter is used for measuring pH in solutions, broth cultures, milk, and milk products.

14. **Spectrophotometer**: A spectrophotometer is a more advanced version of a colorimeter that uses monochromatic light, usually from a prism, to measure the absorption of specific wavelengths, including those in the UV range (below 360 nm). Key components include:
    i) **Source**: A deuterium lamp for UV light and a tungsten lamp for visible light.
    ii) **Monochromator**: A prism used for resolving shorter wavelengths.
    iii) **Cell Compartment**: Holds cuvettes made of glass for visible light and quartz for UV light.
    iv) **Photoelectric Device**: Converts light energy into electrical energy.
    v) **Measuring Device**: Directly measures the percentage of transmittance or optical density.
15. **Centrifuge**: A centrifuge is used for separating solids from liquids or microbial cells from the liquid phase. Different types include:
    i) **Desk Top Centrifuge**: Small and simple, used for rapidly sedimenting substances like red blood cells or yeast cells, with a maximum speed of 3,000 rpm.
    ii) **High-Speed Centrifuge**: Can reach speeds of up to 25,000 rpm and provides centrifugal forces up to 90,000 g. These centrifuges are equipped with cooling systems to regulate temperature between 0-40°C.
    iii) **Ultra Centrifuge**: Operates at speeds up to 75,000 rpm, generating forces up to 500,000 g. It is used for isolating subcellular organelles and features an evacuated rotor chamber and temperature control between 0-4°C.

2

Washing and Cleaning in Microbiology Lab

1. Introduction

All glassware used for bacteriological work must be meticulously cleaned and sterilized. Used and soiled glassware should be thoroughly washed to remove dirt and solid residues before drying and undergoing sterilization.

2. Cleaning of New Glassware

Borosilicate glass (e.g., Pyrex) and factory-washed soda glass require only standard washing before use. However, new, unwashed soda glass needs additional treatment to neutralize alkali content.

- Place the items (e.g., test tubes, Petri dishes, and flasks) in a suitable container, cover with a 1% tri-sodium phosphate solution, and bring to a boil.
- Remove the items, rinse with tap water, and immerse them in a 1% hydrochloric acid solution to neutralize alkalinity.
- Rinse thoroughly with tap water, followed by distilled water. Allow the glassware to dry before sterilization.

3. Cleaning of Used Glassware and Other Apparatus

- Autoclave all glassware contaminated by microorganisms (121°C for 15–20 minutes). This liquefies solid media, facilitating removal.
- Rinse the empty glassware with tap water, then warm water (50–55°C).
- Soak in a detergent solution (e.g., 1% washing soda or tri-sodium phosphate solution) and scrub with a brush.
- Rinse thoroughly with tap water to remove detergent traces, followed by distilled water.
- Drain and dry in a heated drying cabinet before sterilization.

4. Cleaning of Used Pipettes

Used pipettes must be immersed in chromic acid solution for 6–8 hours to remove organic residues like fats and proteins.

- **Preparation of Chromic Acid Solution**: Dissolve 80 g of potassium dichromate in 300 mL of water. Slowly add 460 mL of concentrated sulfuric acid while stirring. Store the solution in large glass bottles.
- As an alternative to chromic acid, 1% potassium permanganate or Lysol solutions can be used for preliminary cleaning.
- After soaking, rinse the pipettes thoroughly with clean water to remove traces of the cleaning solution. Allow them to drain and dry.

5. Cleaning of Microscopic Slides and Cover Slips

Slides require careful cleaning to ensure they are grease-free for proper staining and smear preparation.

- Immerse slides in hot chromic acid solution for several hours.
- Wash thoroughly with clean water, then drain and dry. Wipe with a clean, grease-free cloth.
- To remove oil, immerse the slides in xylene before washing.
- Store cleaned slides and cover slips in 50% alcohol in bottles or jars until use.

Questions

1. Why are pipettes immersed in chromic acid solution before cleaning?
2. How would you remove oil from slides?

3

Sterilization and Sanitization in Microbiology Lab

Introduction

Sterilization of culture media, containers, and instruments is crucial in bacteriological work to ensure the isolation and maintenance of pure cultures. Sterilization and sanitization are essential processes in a microbiology lab to prevent contamination and ensure accurate results. **Sterilization** refers to the complete elimination of all microorganisms, including bacteria, fungi, viruses, and spores, using methods like autoclaving, dry heat, filtration, and chemical agents. **Sanitization**, on the other hand, reduces microbial load to a safe level through cleaning and disinfection using alcohols, detergents, and UV light. These practices maintain aseptic conditions, protect lab personnel, and preserve sample integrity. Proper sterilization and sanitization are fundamental to microbiological research, clinical diagnostics, and industrial applications, ensuring reliable and reproducible experimental outcomes.

Preparations for Sterilization

Before sterilization, cleaned and dried test tubes and flasks should be carefully plugged with clean, non-absorbent cotton. Pipettes should also be plugged at the mouth end, and the plugs should remain in place during use to minimize oral contamination. Cotton plugs provide sufficient ventilation for bacterial growth while preventing external contamination.

To prepare a cotton plug

- Take a square piece of cotton, fold it once on all sides, and roll it into a plug that fits the container.

For glass-stopper bottles, place a piece of paper between the bottle and stopper before sterilization to prevent jamming. Below are the various sterilization techniques:

1. Sterilization by Heat

Heat sterilization is the most reliable and widely used method. Moist heat is generally more effective than dry heat, but both have specific applications.

a) **Dry Heat Sterilization:** Dry heat works by denaturing proteins and oxidizing essential cell components:

i) Flaming

- Used for materials like inoculating needles, wires, and scalpel tips by holding them in a flame until red hot.
- Also used for sterilizing the mouths of culture tubes and cotton plugs during culture transfer.
- Dipping or swabbing in alcohol followed by flaming is effective for sterilizing tools like spatulas, scalpels, and mortars.

ii) Hot Air Oven

- Suitable for dry glassware such as test tubes, Petri plates, flasks, and pipettes.
- Place items in appropriate containers (e.g., stainless steel racks) and sterilize at 160–180°C for 2–2.5 hours.

Precautions

1. Avoid overheating to prevent charring of cotton plugs.
2. Cool items inside the oven for at least 2 hours to avoid breakage.
3. Ensure sufficient air circulation for uniform sterilization.

b) **Moist Heat Sterilization:** Moist heat is effective at lower temperatures, killing microorganisms by denaturing their enzymes and proteins.

i) Autoclaving

- Autoclaving uses high-pressure saturated steam at 121°C (15 psi) for 15–20 minutes.
- Suitable for culture media, fluids, and contaminated items.
- Place items above the water level in the autoclave and ensure proper closure of the lid.

Precautions

1. Ensure the autoclave is sealed properly to prevent leakage.
2. Remove all air from the chamber before starting sterilization.
3. Regulate time and pressure according to the material being sterilized.

2. Sterilization by Filtration

This method is used for heat-sensitive materials like serum, antibiotic solutions, and urea.

- **Seitz Filtration:** Sterilize the assembly, then filter the material aseptically using a vacuum pump.

- **Membrane Filtration:** Use a cellulose acetate membrane with a pore size of 0.22 µm for sterilization. Sterilize the setup beforehand and collect the filtrate in sterilized containers.

Applications include carbohydrate solutions, alcohol, salt solutions, vitamins, and water.

3. Intermittent Steam Sterilization

Used for heat-sensitive media like sugar, gelatin, and milk.

Methods

- **Single heating:** Heat at 100°C for 90 minutes.
- **Tyndallization:** Heat at 100°C for 30 minutes on three consecutive days, with incubation at room temperature between heatings to destroy germinated spores.

4. Sterilization by Chemicals

Chemical disinfectants are used for sterilizing surfaces, articles, and materials that cannot withstand heat.

- **Disinfectants:** Lysol, phenol, bleaching powder, hypochlorite solutions (5–10%), and formalin.
- **Skin Antiseptics:** Iodine tincture and 70% alcohol.
- **Formalin (40% formaldehyde):** Used for instrument sterilization.

Questions

1. Explain the principle by which glassware and different media are sterilized.
2. What is the advantage of using cotton plugs for test tubes and flasks?
3. How do you sterilize saline water?
4. When are bacterial filters used for sterilization?
5. How do you sterilize rubber bands and Bakelite caps?
6. How do you sterilize the following: blood serum, media, milk, sugar media, saline water, laboratory benches, and platinum wires?

4

Basics of Microscopy

A. Construction, Use and Care of Light Microscope

Introduction

Microorganism are invisible to naked eyes, hence their detailed study requires a microscope. A microscope can be defined as an optical instrument consisting of a lens or a combination of lenses for getting enlarged or magnified images of minute objects. A simple microscope is essentially an ordinary magnifying lens held on an adjustable stand. Usually it gives magnification up to 20 times the size of the object. A compound microscope consists of two separate lens system – the objective and the eye piece. It gives much greater magnification (100-1500 times) than a simple microscope and is, therefore useful for viewing and examining very minute objects like protozoa, bacteria, yeast, mold and algae which cannot be seen with naked eyes.

The objective of this exercise is to familiarize the students with construction and the use of compound light microscope.

1. Construction of Microscope

A microscope contrite various parts in which principle parts are described below:

i) **Frame work:** All microscopes have a basic frame structure which includes the arm and base. All other parts are attached to this framework and the base support the microscope.

ii) **Stage:** It is a horizontal platform that supports the microscopic slide. It has a mechanical stage, which is used for holding and moving the slide around on the stage.

iii) **Body Tube:** Through this, the light passes from the objective to eyepiece. The initial magnifications worked on the objectives are for a standard tube length i.e. 160-170 mm.

Parts of the Light Microscope

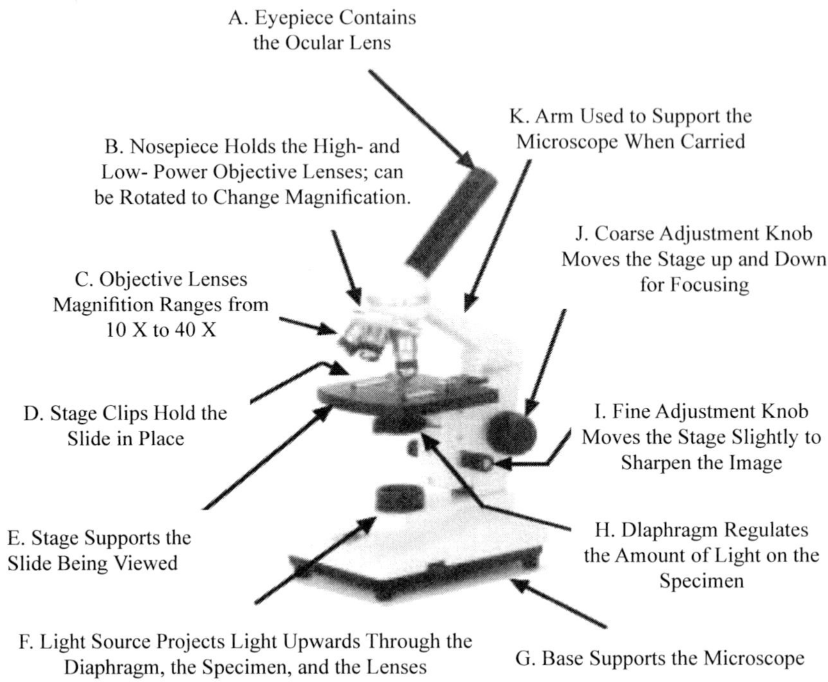

Fig.: Parts of Light Microscope

iv) **Light Source and Mirror:** In the base of most microscopes there is a built in a light source such as lamps with adjustable light intensity. Light passes directly into the condenser and mirror is not required in such microscope. In case, where such facility is not available a mirror is provided for reflecting the light source into the condenser. Mirror is usually double mirror having one side plane and the other concave. Concave side is particularly used for artificial light.

v) **Lens Systems:** All microscopes have three lens systems the ocular, the objectives and the condenser.

vi) **Ocular for Eye Piece:** It is at the top of the instrument, consisting of two or more internal lenses and usually has a magnification of 10X or 50X. The images seen by the eye has a total magnification equal to the product of magnification objective and eye piece. A binocular body, having two parallel tubes with similar eye pieces is also fitted in the microscopes which permits the use of both the eyes and give some appearance of depth of image.

vii) **Objectives:** There or more objectives are usually used which are attached to a rotatable nose pieces which make it possible to move them into position over a slide. Objectives on most laboratory microscope have magnification of 10X, 45X, and 100X designed as low power, high dry and oil immersion respectively. The objective lens system is placed just over the specimen or object to be viewed.

Oil immersion objective is most frequently used because of its greater magnification and resolution. Cedar wood oil with the same refractive index (1.515) is that of glass is used as immersion oil so that the light can pass as homogeneous path of light directly into the objective without refraction.

viii) **Condenser:** This is third lens system which is located under the stage. It collects and directs the light from the lamp to the slide being studied.

ix) **Sub Stage Adjustment Knob:** This knob enables to move the condenser up and down for regulating the intensity of light coming to the object.

x) **Iris Diaphragm:** This controls the amount of light exiting from the condenser under the stage.

xi) **Focusing Knob:** Used for bringing objects into focus

xii) **Coarse Adjustment Knob:** This is a screw mechanism by which either the body tube with lens system or the stage can be raised or lowered to bring the object approximately into focus.

xiii) **Fine Adjustment Knob:** This has limited range and it is used to bring the object exactly into focus after the coarse adjustment is made.

2. Use of the Microscope

i) Hold the microscope with both the hands and place it on the laboratory bench firmly. Wipe dust from the microscope especially from eye piece and mirror.

ii) Place the microscope lamp at a suitable distance from the microscope and adjust the concave side of the mirror against the lamp such that it reflects and throw a bright beam of light on the object, when indirect sunlight is used turn the plain mirror towards it so as to reflect maximum light on the object.

iii) Position the side on the stage with material to be studied on the upper surface of the slide. Hold the slide in place by the mechanical stage retainer lever.

iv) Turn on light and position the stained material exactly on the center on the light source.

v) Raised the condenser to its highest point.

vi) Sowing the low power objective into position and lower the tube to bring the objective about 1/4 inches above the slide. Look through the eye piece and adjust the opening of the iris diaphragm and the position of the mirror to obtain uniformly lighted field.

vii) Turn the coarse adjustment knob to lower the objective until it stop. A built-in stop will prevent the objective from touching the slide.

viii) While looking down through the ocular or oculars, bring the object into focus by turning the fine adjustment focusing knob. Don't readjust the coarse adjustment knob.

ix) Manipulate the diaphragm lever to reduce or increase the light intensity to produce the clearest and sharpest image.

x) Once the image is visible, move the slide by turning the knobs that move the mechanical stage and note the size and shape of the cells.

xi) Swing the high power dry objective (45X) into position. If a microscope is of good quality, only mirror focusing adjustments are needed when changing from low power to high power because all the objectives will be parfocalized. In non-parfocalized microscope considerable focusing adjustments are required.

xii) Lower the objective until it almost touches the slide (take care that lens does not touch the slide). Increase the brightness of field by bringing the condenser very close to the slide. Then slowly raise the objective and focus using the coarse and fine adjustment knobs. Observe the size and appearance of the cells.

xiii) Place a drop of cedar wood oil on the stained area. Swing the oil immersion objective into line. Carefully lower the objective until its tip enters oil and almost touches the slide. Looking through ocular and using the coarse adjustment raise the tube slowly until cells come into focus. Always focus while raise the tube, never while lowering it, sharper the focus with the fine adjustment knob. Adjust the amount of light to give adequate illumination. Observe the size and appearance of the cells.

3. Returning Microscope to Cabinet

After completing the observations, return the microscope to the cabinet following these steps:

1. Remove the slide from the stage.
2. If immersion oil has been used wipe it off with the lens with xylene and lens paper and with dry lens paper.

3. Rotate the low power objective into position.
4. Adjust the mechanical stage so that it does not project too far on either side.
5. Return the microscope to its correct place in the cabinet.

4. Care of Microscope

Microscopes represent considerable expenses and can be damaged rather easily if certain precautions are not observed.

The following precautions should be taken while handling a microscope:-

i) Use both hands when holding the instrument. Otherwise there is always chance of collision with furniture or some other object.

ii) Do not remove any part of microscope.

iii) The coarse and fine adjustment knobs should always be done by first lowering the objective to come very near the slide and then slowly raising it.

iv) While lowering the objective for focusing take care that it does not press on the slide. If you are careless the slide will be broken and may be damaged.

v) It is a good practice to keep both eyes open while looking through the eye piece.

vi) Keep the lenses free of dust, oil and other contaminants. Clear the oil immersion lens with lens paper using minimum amount of xylene. Wipe off the entire lens before keeping the microscope in the box.

vii) Clean the ocular with lens paper on top lens and for lower lens, clean with lens paper and blowing off with air syringe.

viii) Wipe off the condenser with lens paper to remove the dust on the top surface of condenser.

ix) Keep the instrument free of dust and moisture.

5. Terminology Used in Microscopy

i) **Resolution:** Resolution is the ability to distinguish between two points; The closer the two points, the higher the resolution. Resolution or resolution power of best microscope is around 0.2 mm. This means that two small objects that are 0.2 mm. apart will be seen as separate entities.

ii) **Magnification:** Relative enlargement of the specimen, the total magnification of the image is calculated by multiplying the magnification of the ocular by the magnification of the objective.

iii) **Depth of Focus:** Thickness of a specimen that can be seen in focus at one time and as magnification increase the depth of focus decrease.

iv) **Field of Vision:** The surface area of view, the area decrease as magnification increase.

v) **Numerical Aperture (N.A.):** The amount of light reaching the specimen, as N.A. increase the resolution increase

B. Overview of Different Types of Electron Microscopes

Electron microscopes are advanced imaging tools that utilize electron beams instead of light to achieve extremely high resolution and magnification, enabling the observation of structures at the molecular and atomic levels. These microscopes play a crucial role in fields such as materials science, biology, and nanotechnology. The two main types of electron microscopes are the **Transmission Electron Microscope (TEM)** and the **Scanning Electron Microscope (SEM)**, each designed for specific imaging applications. In addition to these, specialized electron microscopes, such as **Scanning Transmission Electron Microscope (STEM)** and **Cryo-Electron Microscope (Cryo-EM)**, have been developed for specific applications, offering enhanced capabilities in imaging and structural analysis. These advanced instruments continue to expand our understanding of the microscopic world.

I. Transmission Electron Microscope (TEM) Overview

A Transmission Electron Microscope (TEM) is a powerful imaging device that uses high-energy electrons to produce detailed, two-dimensional images of thin specimens. TEM is particularly valuable for studying the internal structure of cells, organelles, and materials at nanometer to atomic resolution.

Key Components and Their Functions

1. Electron Gun

- Located at the top of the TEM, the electron gun generates a high-energy electron beam.
- **Components**
    - **Cathode (Filament):** Often tungsten, it emits electrons when heated.
    - **Anode:** Accelerates electrons toward the specimen.
- The accelerating voltage typically ranges from 60–300 kV.

2. Condenser Lenses

- Electromagnetic lenses that focus the electron beam onto the specimen.
- Ensure uniform illumination of the sample.

3. Specimen Stage

- A platform that holds the ultra-thin sample (approximately 50–100 nm thick) in place.
- Often allows for tilting and rotation to observe the specimen from different angles.

4. Objective Lens

- The most critical lens in the TEM system, it magnifies and focuses the electrons passing through the specimen.
- Creates the first intermediate image.

5. Projector Lenses

- Further magnify the image formed by the objective lens.
- Transmit the magnified image to the imaging system.

6. Vacuum System

- The TEM operates under a high vacuum to prevent electrons from scattering due to collisions with air molecules.

7. Fluorescent Screen

- Displays the image formed by electrons exiting the sample.
- Used for real-time observation of the sample.

8. Digital Detector (or Camera)

- Captures and records electron micrographs digitally.

9. Electron Diffraction Unit (Optional)

- Used to analyze the crystalline structure of materials by observing diffraction patterns.

Working Principle

1. Electrons are emitted from the electron gun and accelerated by the anode.
2. The condenser lenses focus the electron beam onto the sample.
3. As electrons pass through the ultra-thin specimen, some are scattered depending on the specimen's density and composition.
4. The unscattered and scattered electrons are magnified by the objective and projector lenses.
5. The magnified image is projected onto a fluorescent screen or captured by a digital camera.

TEM enables visualization of fine details, such as organelles in cells or atomic arrangements in crystals, with resolutions up to 0.1 nm. Its ability to provide both images and diffraction patterns makes it indispensable in research and diagnostics.

II. Scanning Electron Microscope (SEM)

Introduction

A Scanning Electron Microscope (SEM) is an advanced imaging tool that uses a focused beam of high-energy electrons to scan the surface of a specimen. Unlike a Transmission Electron Microscope (TEM), which provides internal structural details, SEM generates three-dimensional (3D) images of surface topography and composition with high resolution and depth of field. SEM is extensively used in materials science, biology, forensics, and nanotechnology.

Working Principle

1. Electron Beam Generation

- A high-energy electron beam is emitted by the electron gun and focused into a narrow beam by electromagnetic lenses.

2. Beam-Specimen Interaction

- The focused beam scans the specimen's surface point by point in a raster pattern.
- When the beam interacts with the sample, various signals are generated, such as secondary electrons, backscattered electrons, and X-rays.

3. Detection

- These signals are captured by detectors, each providing specific information:
  - **Secondary Electrons (SE):** Produce images of surface topography.
  - **Backscattered Electrons (BSE):** Provide compositional contrast.
  - **X-rays:** Reveal elemental composition through Energy-Dispersive X-ray Spectroscopy (EDS).

4. Image Formation

- The detected signals are processed and converted into high-resolution images of the specimen's surface.

Components of SEM

1. Electron Gun

- Generates the electron beam.
- Common types include thermionic emitters (e.g., tungsten filament) and field emission guns (FEG).

2. Electromagnetic Lenses

- **Condenser Lenses:** Focus the electron beam into a fine spot.
- **Objective Lenses:** Further refine the beam for interaction with the sample.

3. Scanning Coils

- Direct and move the electron beam across the specimen in a raster pattern.

4. Specimen Chamber

- Contains the sample on a stage that can be adjusted for rotation, tilt, and height.
- Maintained under high vacuum conditions to ensure electron beam stability.

5. Detectors

- **Secondary Electron Detector:** Produces images based on surface morphology.
- **Backscattered Electron Detector:** Detects atomic number contrast.
- **X-ray Detector:** Used for compositional analysis.

6. Vacuum System

- Maintains a vacuum environment to minimize scattering and ensure uninterrupted electron flow.

7. Display and Control System

- Processes signals from detectors and displays the resulting image on a computer screen.

Applications of SEM

- Surface morphology studies of materials.
- Compositional analysis using EDS.
- Failure analysis in engineering.
- Examination of biological specimens, often after coating with a conductive layer.

Advantages of SEM

- High resolution and depth of field.
- Ability to analyze surface details and composition.
- Versatility across diverse fields of study.

By leveraging its 3D imaging capabilities and compositional analysis, SEM is a critical tool for scientific research and industrial applications.

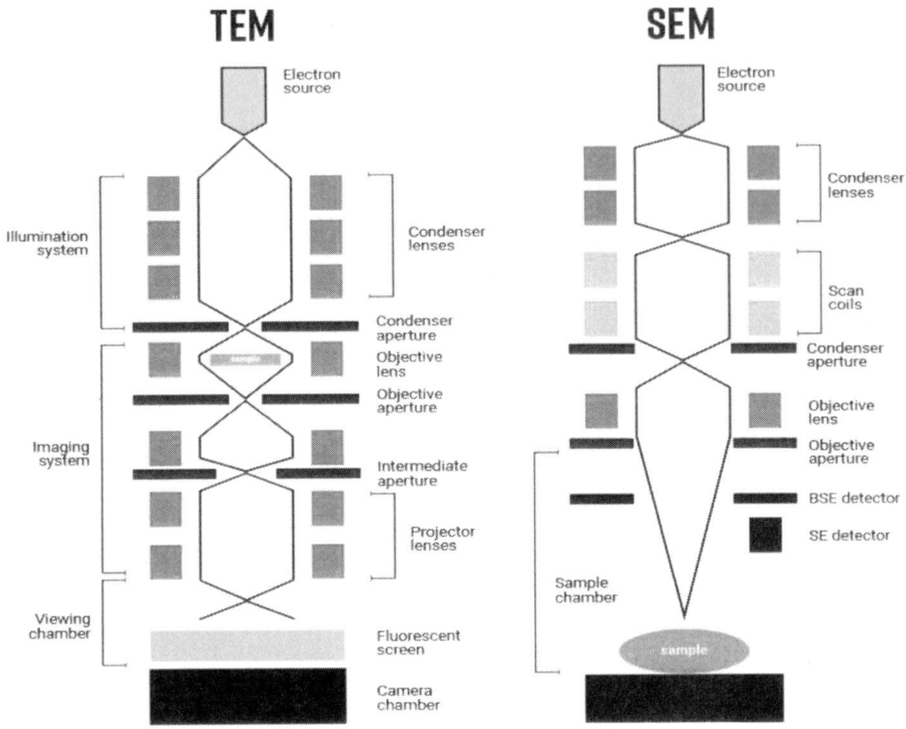

Fig. : Schematic diagram of TEM vs SEM (Courtesy: https://www.nanoscience.com)

Questions

1. What is the difference between a simple and compound microscope?
2. Why cedar wood oil is used with oil immersion lens?
3. What is the maximum magnification in a compound microscope?
4. What types of objectives and eye pieces are present in a compound microscope?
5. What care is necessary regarding the maintenance of the microscope lenses? Why?
6. List three fluids that may be used for cleaning lenses?
7. How the diaphragm functions?
8. What is the maximum resolution of the compound microscope in terms of micrometer?

C. Different Types of Microscope

Introduction

- On the basis of source of illumination and types of lenses used, microscopes can be broadly categorized into:
  - **Light Microscopes**– Use visible light as a source of illumination and optical lenses as magnifying objects.
  - **Electron Microscopes**–Use electrons (electron beam) and electromagnetic lenses for magnifying objects.
  - On the basis of working, microscopes are classified as:
  - **Simple Microscope**–Only a single lens is used for magnifying objects. These do not have high magnification. Example, handheld magnifying glass.
  - **Compound Microscope**–Use multiple lens systems for magnifying objects. These have higher magnification. Example, bright-field compound microscope.

1. Light Microscopes

Microscopes using visible light can be categorized into following types:

i) Bright-field microscope

ii) Dark-field microscope

iii) Phase-contrast microscope

iv) Fluorescence microscopes

All these applications employed in compound microscopes which are described below:-

i) Bright Field Microscope

- The bright-field light microscope is an instrument that magnifies images using two-lens systems. Initial magnification occurs in the objective lens.
- Most microscopes have at least three objective lenses on a rotating base, and each lens may be rotated into alignment with the eye piece or ocular lens in which the final magnification occurs.

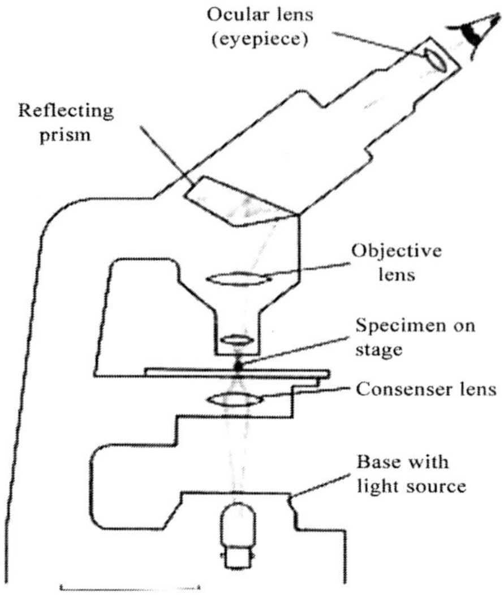

Fig. : Bright Field Microscope

- The objective lenses are identified as the low-power (10X, 16mm), high-dry (40X, 4mm), and oil immersion (100X, 1.8mm) objectives. Here, 10X is the magnifying power of the lens and 16mm is the focal length.
- As the magnification increases, the size of the lens at the tip of the objective becomes progressively smaller and admits less light. This is one of the reasons that changes in position of the sub-stage condenser and iris diaphragm are required when using different objectives if the specimens viewed are to be seen distinctly.
- When the oil immersion lens is used, immersion oil fills the space between the objective and the specimen. Because immersion oil has the same refractive index as glass, the loss of light is minimized.
- The eyepiece, or ocular, at the top of the tube magnifies the image formed by the objective lens. As a result, the total magnification seen by the observer is obtained by multiplying the magnification of the objective lens by the magnification of the ocular, or eyepiece. For example, when using the 10X ocular and the 40X objective, total magnification is $10 \times 40 = 400$ times.

ii) Dark Field Microscope

- When compound microscope is fitted with a dark-field condenser that has a numerical aperture (resolving power) greater than the objective. It acts as a dark-field microscope.

- Light passing through the specimen is diffracted and enters the objective lens, whereas undiffracted light does not, resulting in a bright image against a dark background.
- Since light objects against a dark background are seen more clearly by the eye than the reverse, dark-field microscopy is useful in observing unstained living microorganisms, microorganisms that are difficult to stain, and spirochetes, which are poorly defined by bright-field microscopy.

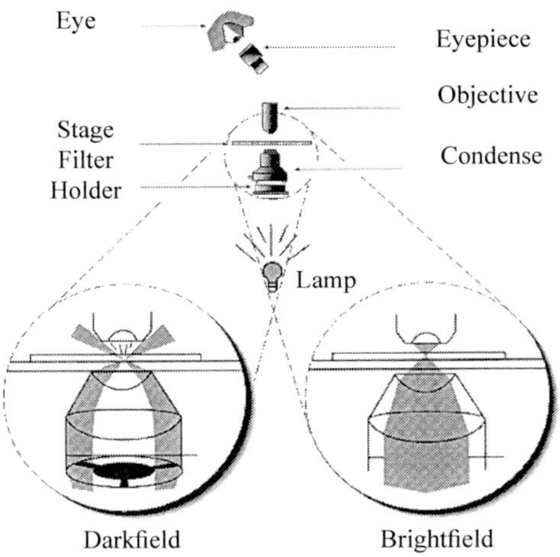

Fig. : Light Path Dark field and Bright field Microscope

iii) Phase Contrast Microscope

- This is first microscopic method which allowed visualization of live cells in action. The Nobel Prize in physics was awarded to Frits Zernike in 1953 for its discovery.
- The phase contrast microscope permits the observation of otherwise invisible living, unstained microorganisms. It enhances contrast in transparent and colorless objects by influencing the optical path of light. It uses the fact that light passing through the specimen travels slower than the undisturbed light beam, i.e. its phase is shifted.
- Phase contrast microscopy effectively converts this phase shift into an intensity difference we can detect.

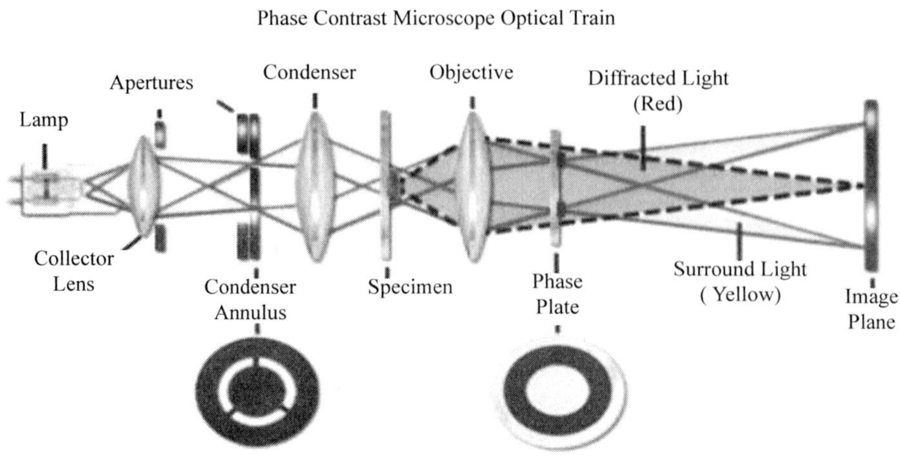

Fig. : Light Path Phase Contrast Microscope

- In the phase contrast microscope, the condenser has an annular diaphragm, which produces a hollow cone of light; the objective has a glass disk (the phase plate) with a thin film of transparent material deposited on it, which accentuates phase changes produced in the specimen. This phase change is observed in the specimen as a difference in light intensity.
- Phase plates may either retard (positive phase plate) the diffracted light relative to the undiffracted light, producing dark phase contrast microscopy, or advance (negative phase plate) the undiffracted light relative to the directed light, producing bright phase contrast microscopy.

iv) Fluorescence Microscope

- A fluorescence microscope is much the same as a conventional light microscope with added features to enhance its capabilities.
- The conventional microscope uses visible light (400-700 nanometers) to illuminate and produce a magnified image of a sample. Whereas, a fluorescence microscope uses a much higher intensity light source which excites a fluorescent species in a sample of interest. This fluorescent species in turn emits a lower energy light of a longer wavelength that produces the magnified image instead of the original light source.

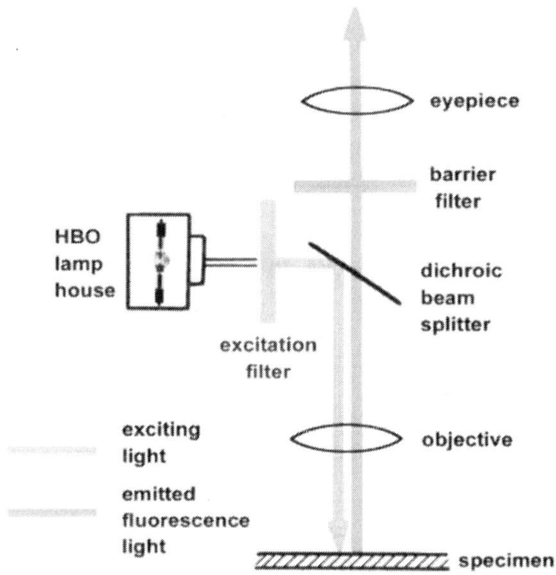

Fig. : Light Path in Fluorescence Microscope

2. Electron Microscopes

- Electron microscopes were developed in order to overcome the limitations of light microscopes, which are constrained by the physics of light to 500X or 1000X magnification and a resolution of 0.2 µm.
- In the early 1930s this theoretical limit had been reached and there was a scientific desire to see the fine details of the interior structures of organic cells (nucleus, mitochondria, etc.). This required 10,000 plus magnification which was just not possible using Light Microscopes.
- Electron microscopes based on their construction and application, are of two types:
  i) The first **Scanning Electron Microscope** (SEM) debuted in 1942 with the first commercial instruments around 1965. SEM functions exactly as an optical scanning device except that they use a focused beam of electrons instead of light to 'scan' the specimen and gain information as to its structure and composition.
  ii) The **Transmission Electron Microscope** (TEM) was the first type of EM to be developed and is patterned exactly on the Light Transmission Microscope except that a focused beam of electrons is used instead of light to 'see through' the specimen. It was developed by Max Knoll and Ernst Ruska in Germany in 1931.

i) Scanning Electron Microscope [SEM]

SEM is patterned after reflecting light microscopes and yield similar information:

- **Topography:** The surface features of an object or 'how it looks', its texture; detectable features limited to a few manometers.

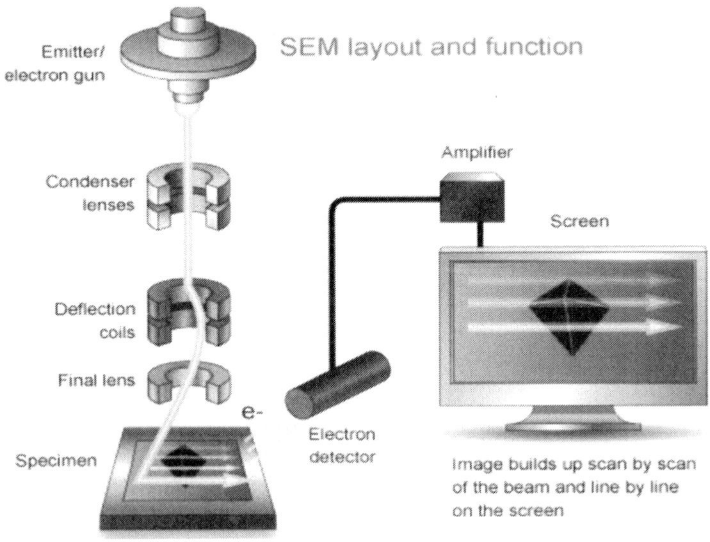

Fig. : SEM Layout

- **Morphology**: The shape, size and arrangement of the particles making up the object that are lying on the surface of the sample or have been exposed by grinding or chemical etching; detectable features limited to a few manometers.
- **Composition:** The elements and compounds the sample is composed of and their relative ratios, in areas ~1 μm in diameter.
- **Crystallographic Information:** The arrangement of atoms in the specimen and their degree of order; only useful on single-crystal particles >20 μm.

Working of SEM

The working of a typical SEM is as follows:

- The 'Virtual Source' at the top represents the electron gun, producing a stream of monochromatic electrons.
- The stream is condensed by the first condenser lens (usually controlled by the 'coarse probe current knob'). This lens is used to both form the

beam and limit the amount of current in the beam. It works in conjunction with the condenser aperture to eliminate the high-angle electrons from the beam.

- The beam is then constricted by the condenser aperture (usually not user selectable), eliminating some high-angle electrons.
- The second condenser lens forms the electrons into a thin, tight, coherent beam and is usually controlled by the 'fine probe current knob'.
- A user selectable objective aperture further eliminates high-angle electrons from the beam.
- A set of coils then 'scan' or 'sweep' the beam in a grid fashion (like a television), dwelling on points for a period of time determined by the scan speed (usually in the microsecond range).
- The final lens, the objective, focuses the scanning beam on the part of the specimen desired.
- When the beam strikes the sample (and dwells for a few microseconds) interactions occur inside the sample and are detected with various instruments.
- Before the beam moves to its next dwell point these instruments count the number of interactions and display a pixel on a CRT whose intensity is determined by this number (the more reactions the brighter the pixel).
- This process is repeated until the grid scan is finished and then repeated, the entire pattern can be scanned 30 times per second

ii) Transmission Electron Microscope (TEM)

TEM are patterned after Transmission Light Microscopes and will yield similar information.

- Morphology: The size, shape and arrangement of the particles which make up the specimen as well as their relationship to each other on the scale of atomic diameters.
- Crystallographic Information: The arrangement of atoms in the specimen and their degree of order, detection of atomic-scale defects in areas a few nanometers in diameter

TEM work the same way except that they shine a beam of electrons (like the light) through the specimen (like the slide). Whatever part is transmitted is projected onto a phosphor screen for the user to see. A more technical explanation of a typical TEM working is as follows:

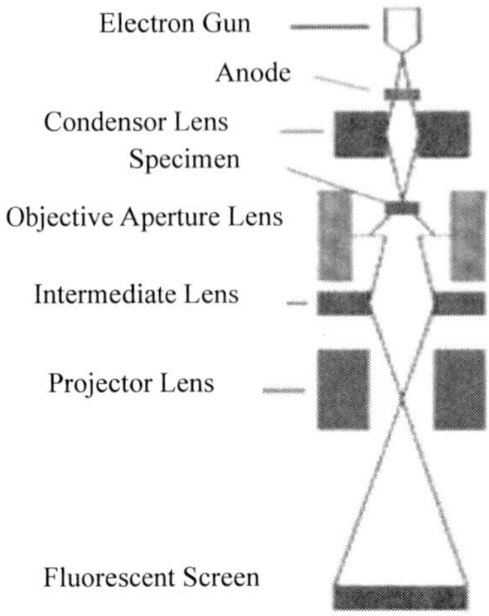

Fig. : Layout of TEM

- The electron gun at the top produces a stream of monochromatic electrons.

This stream is focused to a small, thin, coherent beam by the use of condenser lenses.

- The beam is restricted by the aperture, knocking out high angle electrons.
- The beam strikes the specimen and parts of it are transmitted.
- This transmitted portion is focused by the objective lens into an image.
- The image is passed down the column through the intermediate and projector lenses, being enlarged all the way.
- The image strikes the phosphor image screen and light is generated, allowing the user to see the image. The darker areas of the image represent those areas of the sample that fewer electrons were transmitted through (they are thicker or denser). The lighter areas of the image represent those areas of the sample that more electrons were transmitted through (these are thinner or less dense).

Questions

1. What is the function of condenser in dark field microscope?
2. What objects are seen by dark field microscope?
3. How the phase contrast microscope functions?
4. What kinds of microorganisms are observed by phase contrast microscope?

5. What is the resolving power of ultra violet microscope?
6. Name some fluorescent substances?
7. What is the principle of fluorescence microscope?
8. Which light is used for fluorescent microscopy?
9. For which organism's fluorescent microscope is used?
10. What is the resolving power of Electron microscope?
11. What is the source of light in Electron microscope?
12. What magnification can be achieved by Electron microscope?

5

Preparation of Smear and Simple Staining Technique

Introduction

Ocular micrometer and stage micrometer are used to measure the size of microorganisms. The Ocular micrometer consists of a circular disk of glass which has graduations engraved on surface. A stage micrometer or objective micrometer has scribed lines on it that are exactly 0.01mm (10 micrometer) apart. Ocular micrometer is calibrated for the objective first. To calibrate the ocular micrometer for a given objective, the two scales are superimposed and determined how many of the ocular gradation coincide with one graduation on the stage micrometer scales. Thus, the distance between the graduations on the ocular micrometer can be determined and so the size of the organism can be determined.

Materials

1. Ocular micrometer
2. Stage micrometer
3. Microscope
4. Stained slides of yeast or bacteria

Procedure

1. Insert the ocular micrometer in the eye piece between the two lenses or below bottom lens. Place the gradations on the upper surface of the glass disk.
2. Place the stage micrometer on the stage and center it exactly over the light source.
3. With the low power (10X) objective in position, bring the graduations at the stage micrometer into focus, using the coarse adjustment knob.
4. Rotate the eye piece to bring the graduation of the ocular micrometer parallel to the stage micrometer.

5. Move the stage micrometer to coincide the lines at one end using low power objective, high power objective or oil-immersion lens whichever is to be calibrated. Note the number of lines of ocular micrometer coincide with one graduation of the stage micrometer.
6. For example-6 ocular division match with one stage micrometer division of 0.01 mm so one space is apart by = 10/6 mm or 1.6 m.
7. Replace the stage micrometer with slides of organisms to be measured.
8. Count the number of divisions of ocular micrometer coincide with the length or width of microbial cell.
9. Multiply this number by the known distance between the graduations (i.e. least count number).
10. Draw neat diagram of stage micrometer and ocular micrometer showing their scale.

Record your observation in the following table –

S. No.	Types of organism	No. of division		Diameter	Measurement			Average
		Length	Width		Length	Width	Diameter	

Result

Interpretation

Questions

1. How will you calibrate ocular micrometer?
2. What is the average size of bacterial and yeast cells?

6

Measurement of Size of Microorganisms By Micrometry

Introduction

- **A cell** is the most basic structural and functional unit of life. These are of two types:
  - i) Prokaryotic cells– Prokaryotes are those cells which lack a membrane bound nucleus and other membrane bound cell organelles. These cells are primitive cells. Examples, bacterial cells, archaeal cells.
  - ii) Eukaryotic cells– Eukaryotes are those cells which have distinct membrane bound organelles. These are advanced cells. Example, animal cells, plant cells, fungi.
- A **microorganisms** (from the Greek: mikros, "small" and organism's, "organism") are those small living organisms which cannot be seen with naked eyes. These are of two types:
  - i) Single cell– Organism made up of a single cell.
  - ii) Multi-cellular– Organism made up of multiple cells.

Shape and Arrangement of Bacterial Cells

- Prokaryotes display following shapes
  - Spherical cells called **Cocci**
  - Cylinders called rods or **Bacilli**
  - Coma shaped called **Vibrio**
  - Spiral shaped called **Spirilli**
  - Corkscrew shaped called **Spirochete**
  - Others: Star, Square
- Bacterial shapes, depending on the organism, can change subtly when cells are growing or existing under different conditions, e.g. a shortening of rods as nutrient concentrations are used up and therefore as growth rates decline.

- Most bacteria are **monomerhic**- they maintain the same shape. Some bacteria do not display a constant shape even during growth in an otherwise unchanging, homogeneous environment. Such bacteria are termed **pleomorphic.**

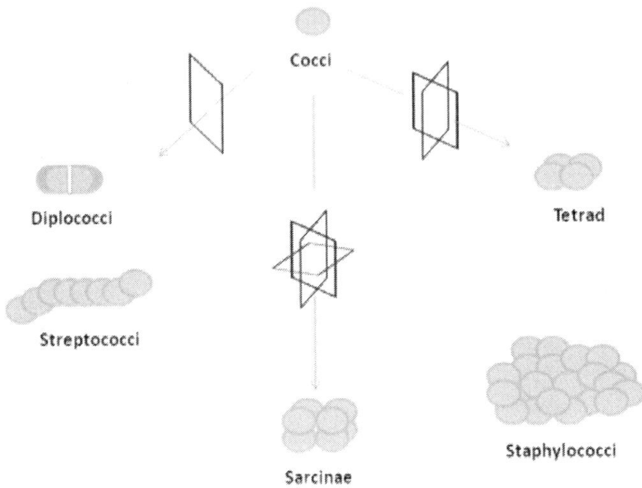

Fig. : Arrangement of Cocci

- Cells are found in distinctive arrangements of group of cells; Occur when cell divide without separating. Cocci can divide in one or more planes leading to different arrangements of cells as follows:-
  - Division in one plane in pairs (**Diplococci**) or in chains (**Streptococci**)
  - Division in two planes: **Tetrads** (4 cells in a cube)
  - Division in 3 planes: **Sarcinae** (8 cells arranged in a cube)
  - Random division: Grape like clusters (**Staphylococci**)
- **Bacilli** divide in one plane (Exception: Bacilli arranged in a rosette attached by stalksto a substrate e.g. Caulobacter and spiral not generally grouped together).

  Like cocci these can be termed as **diplo** and **streptobacilli.**

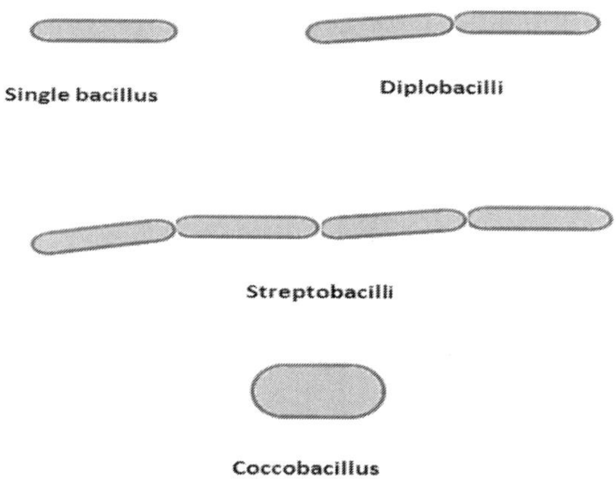

Fig. : Arrangement of Bacilli

I. Smear Preparation

Introduction

In order to observe microstructure such as flagella, granules and endospores specific bacteriological stains are applied. A drop of culture is spread on a glass slide to from a thin film or smear. A properly prepared bacterial smear is one that with stands one or more washing during staining without loss of organisms; smear is not too thick, and does not result in excessive distortion due to shrinkage of cell. Smear is prepared from liquid or solid media.

A. Preparation of Smear from Liquid Culture and Milk

Materials

1. Microscope
2. Glass Slides
3. Inoculating needle
4. Marker
5. Raw milk
6. Broth culture/Sample

Procedure

1. Take a clean, dry and grease free, slides for making a good smear. Pass the slides through the flame two or three times to make it grease free.
2. Heat the platinum wire in the flame and allow it to cool down. Transfer a loopful of the well shaken raw milk or broth culture or suspension of the cells in water, to the slides and spread evenly to get a thin and uniform smear.
3. Air dry the smear and heat fix it by passing through the flame two or three times. Do not heat the slides too much, otherwise smear will burst and disintegrate.

B. Preparation of smear from solid media such as nutrient agar, blood agar etc.

Procedure

1. Place a loopful of water on a clean, grease free slide using a platinum loop.
2. Flame the inoculating needle. Raise the top of the petri plates under aseptic conditions. Cool the inoculating needle by touching a part of the agar having no bacterial growth and touch the tip of the loop on the colony. Transfer the bacteria on the tip of needle to drop of water on the slide. Emulsify the bacterial suspension and spread it evenly to from a thin smear.
3. Allow the smear to air dry and heat fix by passing through the flame rapidly two or three times.

II. Simple Staining

Introduction

Staining is an auxiliary technique used in microscopic techniques used to enhance the clarity of the microscopic image. Stains and dyes are widely used in the scientific field to highlight the structure of the biological specimens, cells, tissues etc.

The use of single stain to color a bacterial organism is simple staining. Some of the most commonly used dyes for simple staining are Methylene blue, Carbol fuchsin and Crystal Violet. These dyes are basic dyes having a positively charged chromophore group. Bacteria are slightly negatively charged hence, have pronounced attraction between cationic chromophores and the organisms.

The staining time for most simple stains is relatively short usually 30 seconds to 2 minutes, depending on the dye affinity. After smear is stained, excess stain is washed off gently, air dried and examined under oil immersion. Such techniques are used for determining basic morphology of micro-organisms.

Materials

1. Methylene blue
2. Crystal violet
3. Carbol fuchsin
4. Slant culture of bacteria (*E.coli, S.lactis, Lb.bulgaricus, and B.subtilis*)
5. Wash bottles
6. Microscope
7. Inoculating needle

Procedure

1. Prepare a thin smear of the bacterial culture on a clean, grease free slide.
2. Place two drops of staining solution (Methylene Blue or Crystal Violet).
3. Retain the stain for

   Methylene Blue - 2-3 minute

   Crystal Violet - 30-45 seconds

   Basic carbol fuchsin - 15-30 seconds

1. After staining the smear remove excess stain by pouring it off and washing the smear with a gentle stream of water.
2. Dry the slides by pressing it with clean blotting paper and air dry the slides.
3. Observe the slide under oil immersion.

Draw a neat diagram of microorganism in the microscopic field.

Culture	Morphology of cell		Remarks
	Shape	Arrangement	
E.coli			
S.lactis			
B. subtilis			
Lb. bulgaricus			
Any other culture			
Milk Sample			
Yeast Culture			

Interpretation

Questions

1. Why are the cells fixed before staining?
2. Give different methods of fixing the smear?
3. How the smear is prepared from a solid medium?
4. Why should bacteria be stained?
5. How do you prepare methylene blue stain?
6. How do you observe a bacterial colony?
7. What are basic dyes, list them?
8. How are basic dyes more successful on bacteria than acidic dyes?

7

Exploration of Negative Staining Method

Introduction

This method consists of mixing the microorganisms in a small amount of India ink or nigrosine and spreading the mixture over a clean slide. These two pigments are not really bacterial stain and do not penetrate the microorganisms. These pigments make the background dark thus making organisms transparent against dark background. This method is useful for determining cell morphology and accurate size as no shrinkage of cells due to heat.

Materials

1. Bacterial culture (*B. subtilis*)
2. Microscopic slides (Clean, Grease Free)
3. Inoculating needle
4. Cedar wood oil
5. Microscope
6. Xylene

Procedure

1. Take a drop of Nigrosine or India ink near the right end of one of the slide.
2. Put the loopful of the culture. Mix it into the drop of India ink or Nigrosine and break up the clumps of bacteria.
3. Place the edge of a spreader slide to the left of the suspension and move the spreader slide towards the suspension until contact is made.
4. Push the spread slide away from the suspension to make a thin smear at the end of spreading stroke.
5. Allow the slide to dry at room temperature. Do not apply heat to the slide.
6. Examine under oil immersion.
7. Draw neat diagram of the morphological features of organisms.

Observation & Results

Questions

1. Write chemical names of the staining agents used for negative staining?
2. What is the advantage of negative staining over simple staining?

8

Exposure to Different Differential Staining Methods Used for Dairy and Food Microbes

A. Gram's Staining

Introduction

The most widely used staining procedure in microbiology is the Gram stain, discovered by the Danish scientist and physician Hans Christian Joachim Gram in 1884. Gram staining is a differential staining technique that differentiates bacteria into two groups: gram-positives and gram-negatives. The procedure is based on the ability of microorganisms to retain color of the stains used during the gram stain reaction. Gram-negative bacteria are decolorized by the alcohol, losing the color of the primary stain, purple. Gram positive bacteria are not decolorized by alcohol and will remain as purple. After decolorization step, a counterstain is used to impart a pink color to the decolorized gram-negative organisms.

The Gram stain procedure enables bacteria to retain color of the stains, based on the differences in the chemical and physical properties of the cell wall.

1. **Gram positive bacteria**: Stain dark purple due to retaining the primary dye called Crystal Violet in the cell wall. Example: *Staphylococcus aureus*
2. **Gram negative bacteria**: Stain red or pink due to retaining the counter staining dye called Safranin

Example

Bordetella pertusis, the causative agent of whooping cough

Salmonella typhi, the causative agent of typhoid

Vibrio cholera, the causative agent of cholera

Escherichia coli, the normally benign, ubiquitous, gut-dwelling bacteria

Gram Stain Mechanism

Structure of Gram Positive Cell Wall

Gram-positive bacteria have a thick mesh-like cell wall which is made up of peptidoglycan (50-90% of cell wall), which stains purple. Peptidoglycan is mainly a polysaccharide composed of two subunits called N-acetyl glucosamine and N-acetyl muramic acid. As adjacent layers of peptidoglycan are formed, they are cross linked by short chains of peptides by means of a transpeptidase enzyme, resulting in the shape and rigidity of the cell wall. The thick peptidoglycan layer of Gram-positive organisms allows these organisms to retain the crystal violet-iodine complex and stains the cells as purple.

Lipoteichoic acid (LTA) is another major constituent of the cell wall of Gram-positive bacteria which is embedded in the peptidoglycan layer. It consists of teichoic acids which are long chains of ribitol phosphate anchored to the lipid bilayer via a glyceride. It acts as regulator of autolytic wall enzymes (muramidases: Bacterial enzymes located in the cell wall that causes disintegration of the cell following injury or death.).

Gram (+) and Gram (-) Cell Walls

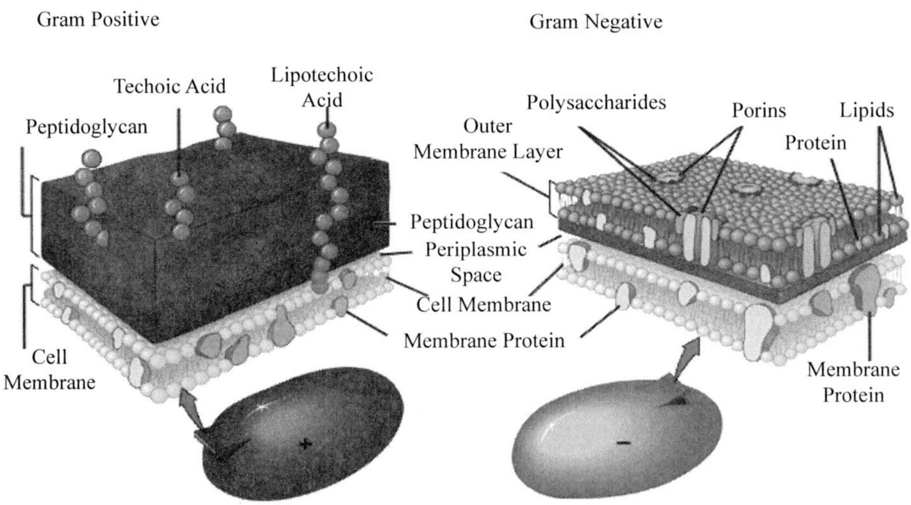

Fig. : Gram Positive and Gram Negative Cell Walls

Structure of Gram Negative Cell Wall

Gram-negative bacteria have a thinner layer of peptidoglycan (10% of the cell wall) and lose the crystal violet-iodine complex during decolorization with the alcohol rinse, but retain the counter stain Safranin, thus appearing reddish or pink. They also have an additional outer membrane which contains lipids, which is separated from the cell wall by means of periplasmic space.

Mechanism of Stain Reactions

The four basic steps of the Gram Stain are described below

1. **Application of the primary stains Crystal Violet (CV) to a heat-fixed smear of bacterial culture:** CV dissociates in aqueous solutions into CV^+ and Cl^- ions. These two ions then penetrate through the cell wall and cell membrane of both Gram-positive and Gram-negative cells. The CV^+ ions later interacts with negatively charged bacterial components and stains the bacterial cells purple.
2. **Addition of Gram's Iodine:** Iodine (I^- or I_3^-) acts as a **mordant** and as a trapping agent. A mordant is a substance that increases the affinity of the cell wall for a stain by binding to the primary stain, thus forming an insoluble complex which gets trapped in the cell wall. In the Gram stain reaction, the crystal violet and iodine form an insoluble complex (CV-I) which serves to turn the smear a dark purple color. At this stage, all cells will turn purple.
3. **Decolorization with 95% Ethyl Alcohol:** Alcohol or acetone dissolves the lipid outer membrane of Gram negative bacteria, thus leaving the peptidoglycan layer exposed and increases the porosity of the cell wall. The CV-I complex is then washed away from the thin peptidoglycan layer, leaving Gram negative bacteria colorless.

On the other hand, alcohol has a dehydrating effect on the cell walls of Gram positive bacteria which causes the pores of the cell wall to shrink. The CV-I complex gets tightly bound into the multi-layered, highly cross-linked Gram positive cell wall thus staining the cells purple.

The decolorization step must be performed carefully, otherwise over-decolorization may occur. This step is critical and must be timed correctly otherwise the crystal violet stain will be removed from the Gram-positive cells. If the decolorizing agent is applied on the cell for too long time, the Gram-positive organisms to appear Gram-negative. Under-decolorization occurs when the alcohol is not left on long enough to wash out the CV-I complex from the Gram-negative cells, resulting in Gram-negative bacteria to appear Gram-positive.

4. **Counterstain with Safranin:** The decolorized Gram negative cells can be rendered visible with a suitable counterstain, which is usually positively charged safranin, which stains them pink. Pink colour which

adheres to the Gram positive bacteria is masked by the purple of the crystal violet (Basic fuschin is sometimes used instead of safranin in rare situations).

Materials

1. Sample or Culture of *Bacillus subtilis, E.coli, Micrococcus sp., Pseudomonas sp., S. lactis.*
2. Crystal Violet
3. Gram's Iodine
4. Ethyl Alcohol (95%).
5. Safranin Solution (0.5% alcoholic).
6. Glass Slides
7. Inoculating needle.
8. Burner.

Procedure

1. Prepare smear of all the culture on clean grease free glass slides.
2. Air dry and heat fix the smears.
3. Cover the smear with crystal violet for 30 seconds.
4. Briefly wash off the stain, using wash bottle of distilled water, drain off excess water.
5. Cover the smear with Gram's iodine solution and let it stand for one minute.
6. Pour off the Gram's iodine and flood the smear with 95% ethyl alcohol for approximately 30 seconds or till the alcohol running out is colorless.
7. Stop the action of alcohol by rinsing the slide with water for a few seconds.
8. Cover the smear with counter stain (safranin) for 20 seconds.
9. Wash gently with water for few seconds, blot with blotting paper and then allow the stained smear to air dry at room temperature.
10. Examine the slide under oil immersion objective.
11. Draw a neat diagram of morphology of microorganisms and label.

Observation Table

S.No.	Sample/Culture	Gram's Reaction	Morphology	Remarks
1.	*B.subtilis*			
2.	*E.coli*			
3.	*Micrococcus* sp.			
4.	*Pseudomonas* sp.			
5.	*S.lactis*			
6.	Any other sample or culture			

Interpretation

Questions

1. What is the role of Gram's iodine in the staining procedure?
2. What is the advantage of Gram's stain over the simple stain?
3. What is the counter stain used in Gram's staining?
4. Give two examples of Gram positive and Gram negative bacteria?
5. Does age of the culture influence Gram's reaction?
6. Group the organisms you know according to Gram's reaction?
7. What part of the bacteria cell (cell wall or protoplast) appears to play the most important role in determining whether or not an organism in Gram-positive?
8. What color would you expect *S.aureus* to be if the iodine step were omitted in the Gram Staining procedure?

B. Spore Staining

Introduction

- The spore (i.e. endospore), discovered in 1876 by Cohn, Koch and Tyndall independently, is one of the hardiest dormant life forms on earth formed during the resting stage in the life cycle of spore-forming bacteria.
- Spores can survive for a very long time, and then re-germinate.
- Bacterial endospores are complex structures whose basic architecture is conserved across species. Endospores enables an organism to resist extreme environmental conditions such as Temperature, Drying, UV radiation, Strong acids and bases, Oxidizing agents, Extremes of both vacuum and ultrahigh hydrostatic pressure.
- The resistance of spore is attributed to following factors:
  - i) The presence of high content of calcium-dipicolinate which stabilizes and protect the DNA
  - ii) DNA-binding proteins protect DNA from heat, drying, chemicals, and radiation
  - iii) Dehydration that results in resistance to heat and radiation
  - iv) DNA repair enzymes are able to repair damaged DNA during germination
- These resistant structures survive heating to 150°C although mostly killed at 121°C in moist medium. They can remain dormant for immense periods of time, perhaps even millions of years.
- Key spore forming genera are ***Bacillus, Clostridium, Sporosarcina, Heliobacterium. Sporosarcinae*** are unique among endospore formers because cells are cocci instead of rods and are strictly aerobic, spherical cells.

Principle of Stain Mechanism

The spores are highly resistant to heat and many chemicals. This resistance to heat and chemicals is due primarily to a thick, tough spore coat. When a spore bearing organism is stained by ordinary dyes the vegetative cell is deeply colored, whereas the spores remain unstained. It is difficult to stain the spores and after the spore takes up the stain it is not easily decolorized. Several methods are available that employ heat to provide stain penetration. The Schaeffer-Fulton and Dorner Methods are principal ones used by most bacteriologists. Scharffer-fulton method is described in this exercise. This method utilized malachite green to stain the endospores and Safranin to stain the vegetative cell.

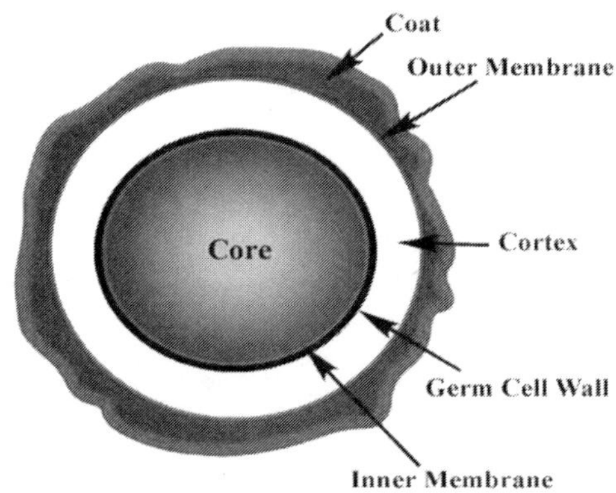

Fig. : Structure of Spore

Materials

1. 24 hr. old culture of *Bacillus subtilis* on nutrient agar slant
2. 5% aqueous solution of Malachite Green
3. 0.5% aqueous solution of safranin
4. Clean slides
5. Inoculating needle
6. Beaker of water
7. Hot plate

Procedure

1. Prepare a smear of the culture, air dry and heat fix the smear
2. Cover the smear with Malachite Green. Steam over boiling water for 5 minutes
3. Add additional stain if it boils off so that stains does not dry up
4. Cool the slide and wash with water for 30 seconds
5. Cover the slide with counter stain (Safranin)
6. Rinse with water to remove excess stain
7. Blot the slide with blotting paper and air dry
8. Examine the slide under oil-immersion, and draw neat diagram and make labeling of your observations

Observation & Results

Interpretation

On the basis spore position in bacterial cell, they can be termed as central, eccentral or terminal spores.

Questions

1. What is the significance of spore in dairy and food industry?
2. How would you demonstrate the presence of spores in milk without spore staining and microscope examination?
3. What is the difference between a vegetative cell and a spore?
4. Where the spores are located in the cell?
5. Give examples of spore formers?
6. Why steaming should be done with malachite green?
7. Why are endospores difficult to stain?

C. Capsular Staining

Introduction

Glycocalyx– It is the term to describe substances that surround bacterial cells.

1. **Capsule:** If substance is organized and firmly attached to cell wall
2. **Slime Layer:** If substance is unorganized and loosely attached to cell wall

Functions of Capsule

- It contribute to virulence of bacteria by preventing phagocytosis by WBC's e.g. *Streptococcus pneumonia, Bacillus anthracis*
- Prevents drying out or desiccation of cell
- Allows bacteria to adhere to various surfaces

Streptococcus mutans - enamel on teeth to cause dental carries

Klebseilla pneumoniae - attaches to respiratory tract

Production of a detectable capsule is often dependent on the composition of the medium and the age of the culture. Some capsules appear to be made of glycoprotein, others contain polypeptide. Special techniques are necessary to stain and visualize the capsules of bacteria. Presence or absence of capsule can be demonstrated by combining negative and simple technique using India ink and crystal violet.

Materials

1. 36-48 hours old culture *Alcaligenes viscosus*
2. India ink
3. Crystal violet
4. Clean glass slide
5. Inoculating needle

Procedure

1. Mix two loopful of the organisms with a small drop of India ink
2. Spread the suspension over slide and air dry
3. Gently heat dry to fix the organism on the slide
4. Stain the smear with crystal violet for one minute
5. Gently wash off the crystal violet with water
6. Dry the slide with blotting paper
7. Examine the slide under oil-immersion

Observation

Interpretation

Bacterial cells are colored dark purple with capsules colorless against the dark background.

Questions

1. List some of the chemical substances that have been identified in bacterial capsules?
2. What relationship is there between capsules and bacterial virulence?

D. Acid Fast Staining

Introduction

Ziehl-Neelsen staining is another differential staining procedure. This technique is used in staining of *Mycobacterium tuberculosis*, *Mycobacterium leprae* and other related Mycobacteria. Acid- fast bacteria are not easily stained but once stained they resist decolorization with acid alcohol. Mycobacteria have been recognized as acid-fast bacilli, due to presence of warlike lipoidal material, the mycolic acid.

The Ziehl-Neelsen method consists of staining the organism with a hot concentrated dye. The dye combines tenaciously with the mycolic acid and resists decolorization with acid. Following decolorization of non-acid-fast material, counter stain methylene blue is added. A properly stained slide of a mixture of acid fast organism and non-acid-fast bacteria will reveal red acid fast rods with bluish non-acid fast bacteria.

Materials

1. Culture of *Staphylococcus aureus* (non-acid-fast), culture of *Mycobacterium* spp.
2. Acid-fast-staining kit (carbol fuchsin, acid alcohol, methylene blue)

3. Hot plate
4. Burner
5. Inoculating needle

Procedure

1. Prepare the smear of culture of *Mycobacteria* and *Staphylococcus aureus* (mixed) on a clean glass slide
2. Cover the smear with strong Ziehl-Neelsen carbol fuchsin, steam over boiling water for 5 minutes. Add additional stain if stain boils off
3. Allow to cool the slide. Decolorize with acid-alcohol for 15-20 seconds
4. Wash with water to stop the action of acid alcohol
5. Counter stain with methylene blue for 30 seconds
6. Remove excess stain by washing with water
7. Blot dry and examine under oil immersion

Observation & Result

Interpretation

Acid fast cells are red in color and non-acid-fast cells are found blue in color after staining.

Question

1. Is the acid-fast Mycobacteria Gram- positive or Gram-negative?
2. For what two diseases is acid-fast staining of paramount importance?
3. What chemical is responsible for acid-fast nature of Mycobacterium?

E. Flagellar Staining

Introduction

The diameter of bacterium flagella is below the limit of resolution of the microscope, and hence flagella are normally not visible. To make flagella visible, it is necessary to increase flagellar diameter by precipitating a coating of dye over their entire length. Leifson's method accomplishes this by using a single staining reagent that utilizes pararosaniline as a staining agent and tannic acid as a mordant.

Materials

1. Broth cultures of *Pseudomonas* sp., *E.coli.*
2. Glass slides.
3. Leifson's flagellar stain (fresh).

Procedure

1. Clean the slide and make it grease free by heating.
2. Suspend loopful of culture in water.
3. Place 2-3 drops of this bacterial suspension at one end of the clean dry slide. Tilt slide to allow the organisms to flow down over the surface of the slide.
4. Allow the smear to completely air dry. Do not apply any heat.
5. Cover the smear with Leifson's stain and leave it on the slide until all the alcohol evaporates.
6. Wash gently to remove the stain from the slide.
7. Counter stain with methylene blue for 1 minute. Wash the slide and air dry it.
8. Allow the stained organisms to air dry. Examine under oil immersion and draw neat diagram.

Observation & Result

Interpretation

Flagella stain red which can be seen against blue black background. Flagella may be polar, peritrichous or amphitrichous in position.

Questions

1. Why the flagella cannot be seen by simple staining?
2. Which staining agent is used for flagella staining?

9

Morphological Characterization of Different Type of Microbial Cultures

A. Morphological Examination of Bacterial Samples

Introduction

Bacteria are most widely distributed, the simplest in morphology, the smallest in size and difficult to identify. They are prokaryotic and a few are photosynthetic. Most bacteria are only 0.5 to 2.0 μm in diameter. Bacteria are generally rod, spherical or curved shaped. Rod shaped bacteria may vary considerably in length, have square round or pointed ends and may be motile or non-motile. The spherical or coccus shaped bacteria may occur single, in pairs in tetrads, in chains or in regular masses. The helical and curved shaped bacteria exist as slender spirochetes, spirillum and bent rods (vibrios).

In this exercise the ubiquitousness of these organisms will be demonstrated in the air and water, on body and in mouth etc.

Materials

1. Petri plates containing nutrient agar
2. Sterile cotton swabs
3. Sterile water blank
4. Tube of nutrient broth
5. Materials for simple staining

Procedure

1. Expose one open petri plates on the floor, laboratory table or out doors for 10 minutes.
2. Moisten a sterile swab by immersing it into a tube of nutrient broth and extracting most of the broth out of it by pressing the swab against the inside wall of the tube.
3. Rub the moistened swab over a part of your body such as fingers or ear teeth etc. or some object such as door knob, telephone mouth piece etc. and return the swab to the tube of broth.

4. Labels the tubes with source of the bacteria.
5. Incubate the plates and tubes at 37^{0}C for 48 hours.
6. Observe the plates for different types of colonies and examine few colonies by simple staining technique.
7. Observe the tubes for the presence of turbidity and examine microscopically by simple staining.
8. Make drawings of the stained preparations showing the shape and arrangement of various bacteria.

Observation & Result

Questions

1. Name few rod shaped bacteria?
2. Write the name of chain forming cocci?
3. Give examples of some curved bacteria?

B. Morphological Examination of Yeast Samples

Yeasts are single cell organisms larger than bacteria and belong to the group of fungi. They reproduce by budding. A bud or blastospore, forms as an outpoching of the parent cell. Bud may separate from the original cell or remain attached. In some yeasts, buds may remain attached to each other to form a pseudohyphae. Yeast also reproduces by formation of spores. Yeasts are commonly found in soil, fruits, food materials including dairy products like butter and cheese. They ferment sugars producing alcohol and carbon dioxide and are important in the brewery and baking industries.

Materials

1. Broth culture of *Saccharomyces cerevesiae*, *Kluveromyces lactis* and *Candida pseudotropicalis*
2. Methylene blue (0.1% aqueous)
3. Microscopic slides
4. Cavity slide
5. Coverslip

Procedure

1. Prepare hanging drop slide of the three cultures. Compare their morphological characteristics as observed under the oil-immersion objectives.
2. Prepare the slides of three cultures by simple staining technique using methylene blue stain.

3. Observe the morphology of all the yeasts under oil immersion objective.
4. Draw the microorganisms showing the presence of buds and pseudo-hyphae, if present.

Observation

S.No.	Cultures	Shape	Budding	Pseudohyphae	Remarks
1.	*S. cerevisiae*				
2.	*K. lactis*				
3.	*C. pseudotropicalis*				
4.	Sample from plate				

Interpretation

C. Morphological Examination of Molds

Molds are saprophytic or parasitic fungi commonly found in soil, water, tools and other environment. They occur in filamentous form and much larger than bacteria. The filaments of Molds are called hyphae which may be septate or aseptate. A mass of intermeshed hyphae as seen microscopically is a mycelium. Molds reproduce by both asexual and sexual means, Mold form characteristic "cottony" colonies on agar medium. Mold colonies differ in color from each other. The identification of Molds is based on surface, back side color, hyphae structure and types of spores.

Materials

1. Mold culture on Sabouraud's agar
2. Microscopic slides
3. Cover glass
4. Lactophenol cotton blue stain
5. Dissecting needles

Procedure

1. Place the uncovered plate on the stage of microscope and examine the edge of a colored colony with the low power objective. Look for hyphal structure and spore arrangement. The white colonies generally lack spores and are difficult to identify.
2. Compare the colony characteristics and spores with the figures given in textbooks.
3. Make a wet mount slide by transferring a small amount of the culture with a dissecting needle to a drop of Lactophenol cotton blue stain on a slide. Cover with the cover glass and examine under low power and high dry objectives. Refer again the figures given in textbooks for identification.
4. Repeat the procedure in different colonies.

Observation & Result

S. No.	Cultures	Hyphae	Asexual	Spores	Microscopic appearance	Remarks
1.						
2.						
3.						
4.						

Interpretation

Questions

1. What is mycelium?
2. What is hypha?
3. How are true yeasts differentiated from false yeasts?
4. What kind of asexual spores are seen in *Penicillium*?
5. What type of hyphae is seen in *Mucor* and *Rhizopus*?
6. What kind of asexual spores are seen in *Mucor* and *Rhizopus*?

D. Morphological Examination of Algae & Protozoa

Introduction

Algae include the entire photosynthetic eukaryotic organism in the kingdom of Protista. Algae may be unicellular colonial or multicellular. The undifferentiated algae structure is often referred to as a thallus. It lacks the stem, root and leaf structures. The organism is universally present where ample moisture favorable temperature and sufficient sunlight exists. Algae are source of agar, carrageenan (stabilizer in cream) and alginic acid.

Protozoa includes all the animals like microorganisms of the kingdom protista. All are single celled organisms. However, some form colonial aggregates. They are able to form cyst, a resistant dormant stage which enables them to survive drought, heat and freezing.

Materials

1. Pond water samples
2. Microscopic slides
3. Cover glass
4. Rubber bulbed pipette
5. Forceps

Procedure

1. Clean the slides and cover glass with soap and water. Rinse thoroughly and dry.
2. Take the sample with the help of pipette from the bottom of the bottle to get maximum number of organisms. Place drop on the slide. Place the cover glass.
3. Take filamentous algae from bottle using forceps. Place small amount of material on the slide. Place the cover glass.
4. Observe under low-power objectives and the high dry objective.
5. Compare the shape and size of microorganisms with reference books.

Observation

Interpretation

Questions

1. How are algae cells different from plant cells?
2. What is the size of protozoa?
3. Name some parasitic protozoa and disease caused by them.
4. Name some economically useful algae.

10

Enumeration of Microbial Cells by Direct Microscopic Count (DMC) Method

Introduction

This method is used to determine the 'total bacterial count' (living and dead organisms) by direct microscopic examination in samples of broth culture, cell suspension and milk. Simple and Gram's staining techniques are used to stain the cells. This method is simple and a rapid. A known volume (0.01 ml) of the sample is spread over a known area ($1 cm^2$) on a glass slide. The sample is allowed to dry; then stained and examined microscopically. The average number of cells per field is determined and is then calculated by applying microscopic factor.

Materials

1. Microscopic slide with one sq. cm. area marked
2. Breed's pipette (0.01 ml)
3. Methylene blue or Newman's stain
4. Culture of *E.coli* or *Bacillus subtilis*

Procedure

1. Measure the diameter of microscopic field with a stage micrometer using oil immersion objective and 10X eye piece.
2. Area of field πr^2.

Determination of microscopic factor (MF)

Average number 'n' of organisms or cells per field

$$= \frac{\text{Number counted}}{\text{No of field counted}}$$

No. of org./cells in 1 cm^2 = MF × n

Since 0.01 ml of sample was spread over 1 cm^2

No. of cells/ml of sample = MF × n × 100

Preparation of Smear

1. Mix the sample thoroughly
2. Draw 0.01 ml of sample with Breed's pipette
3. Transfer carefully exactly 0.01ml of the sample to the marked area of the slide then spread it evenly over the area using wire loop.
4. Air dry the smear or in incubator at 55°C
5. Stain with methylene blue/ Newman's stain
6. Wash off excess stain gently with water
7. Air dry the stained smear
8. Examine using oil immersion objective

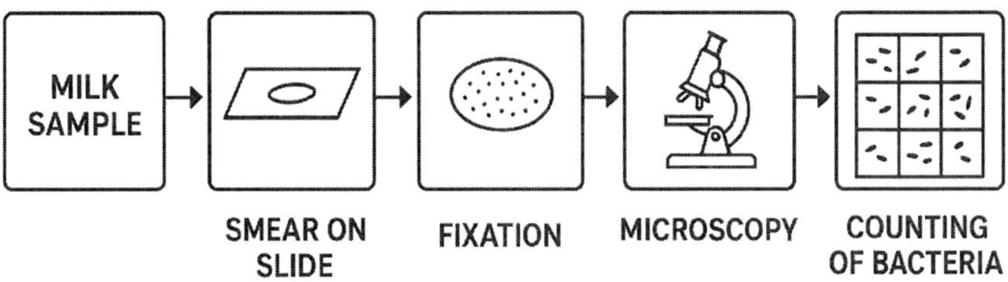

Fig. : Diagram for DMC

Count each single bacterium as one and chains clumps of bacterium as one.

No. of	No. of fields to be counted
0.5	50
0.5-1	25
10-30	5

If the total number of organisms or clumps exceeds 30 per field prepare new smear after making necessary dilution of the sample.

Use Newman's stain if the culture suspension contains fatty materials.

Observation & Result

Questions

1. What is meant by microscopic factor?
2. Compare the direct microscopic count and plate count methods of enumeration of bacteria.

3. What is stage micrometer?
4. How do you calculate the area of a microscopic field?
5. Why are direct counts higher than standard plate counts?

11

Testing of Motility in Bacteria

Introduction

Some species of rod shaped bacteria e.g. *E.coli*, *Ps. fluorescence*, *Bacillus subtilis* are known to be motile. Bacterial motility is generally associated with the presence of hair-like appendages called "Flagella". There are several ways for determining the motility of a culture such as the wet mount method, hanging drop method and a culture method (on semisolid medium). Bacterial cells in suspension also exhibit a vibratory or oscillatory movement without changing their relative position. This is termed 'Brownian Movement' and it should not be confused for true motility of bacteria. In motility the cells change their relative position and move across the microscopic field in different directions.

1. The Wet Mount Technique

This is the simplest and quickest way to determine the motility of bacteria.

Materials

1. Clean glass slide
2. Broth culture of bacteria (*E.coli, Ps.fluroscenes*)
3. Cover glass

Procedure

1. Place a drop of organisms on clean glass slide and cover with a cover glass.
2. Examine the slide with phase contrast microscope or bright field microscope with reduced light under oil-immersion.

Interpretation

Motile organisms are seen moving about. More accurate shape and arrangements of cell is seen because no heat treatment is given in this technique. Heat drying of a smear tends to cause organisms to coalesce.

2. Hanging Drop Method

In this method organisms are observed in a drop that is suspended under a cover glass in a cavity slide.

Materials

1. Depression slides
2. Cover slide
3. Inoculating needle
4. Nutrient broth cultures of organisms (young cultures) of *E.coli, B.subtilis, Ps. fluroscenes* etc.
5. Vaseline or oil.

Procedure

1. Place a very small amount of vaseline near each corner of a cover glass.
2. Place a small drop of culture on the cover glass.
3. Press the depression slide against vaseline on cover glass and quickly invert it so that drop should hang.
4. Examine the slide under low power high dry and then oil immersion objectives.

Observation & Result

Culture	Age of culture	Motility	Remarks
E.coli			
B.subtilis			
Ps. fluorescence			

Interpretation

3. Culture Method (Semisolid Medium)

Slide technique (hanging drop method and wet mount) are not safe for hanging pathogenic microorganisms such as typhoid bacilli, etc. A much safer method is to culture the organisms in a special medium that can demonstrate the presence of motility. In this method, a tube of semisolid medium is inoculated with test organisms by stab technique and examined for cloudiness around the stab after incubation of 24 hours.

Materials

1. Tube of Semi solid medium for motility

2. Nutrient broth of test organisms
3. Inoculating needle (straight)
4. Burner

Procedure

1. Flame and cool the inoculating needle and insert into the culture aseptically.
2. Stab the semisolid medium up to $2/3^{rd}$ of its length with test culture aseptically.
3. Incubate at 37°C for 24 hours.
4. Examine for the presence of cloudiness around the stab.
5. Semisolid media allow the movement of organisms.

Interpretation

Cloudiness seen around the stab shows the migration of motile bacteria from point of inoculation.

Questions

1. What is Brownian movement? How do you distinguish it from bacterial motility?
2. What is the function of flagella in bacterial cells?
3. Name of different types of bacteria according to the position of flagella?
4. What is the effect of age of the culture on motility of bacteria?
5. Which of the two organisms exhibited true motility of the slides?

12

Introduction to Different Types of Culture Media and Their Preparation

Introduction

The characteristics of bacteria used in the study and identification of bacteria depend upon the behavior of populations or cultures rather than of individual organisms. Nutrient materials provided in a form, suitable for growth, are known as culture media. A **Growth Media** or culture medium is a liquid or gel designed to support the growth of microorganisms or cells.

I. Types of Culture Media

Different types of culture media may be used for cultivation of microorganisms such as liquid, solid and semi-solid.

i) **Liquid Culture Media:** Includes nutrient broth, Glucose broth, litmus milk etc. these media are used for the preparation of large number of microorganisms, fermentation studies and various other tests.

ii) **Solid Media:** A little agar, gelatin or silica gel; is added to a liquid medium to impart a degree of firmness to it. Nutrient agar, Blood agar, etc. are examples of solid media that are used for developing surface colony growth of bacteria and mold.

iii) **Agar Slant Media:** Test tubes or small bottles containing about 5ml. of solid medium, e.g. nutrient agar, dissolved and allowed to cool in a sloping position.

iv) **Stab Media:** Tubes or bottles containing agar medium are allowed to solidify in the upright position.

v) **Semi solid Media:** These are more jelly like due to lower percentage of the solidifiers. These media are particularly used for determining motility of bacteria.

Composition of Media

The following factors have important role in constituting culture media: Water, carbon, energy, nitrogen, minerals, growth factors and pH.

i) **Water:** The quantity of water used in preparing media is important. Hard tap water, high in calcium and magnesium ions, should not be used. Always use distilled water.

ii) **Carbohydrates:** Carbohydrates are utilized by bacteria as a source of carbon and energy. Simple sugars are incorporated in many culture media. The property of sugar fermentation is used to differentiate and identify the bacteria.

iii) **Nitrogen:** Autotrophic organisms utilize inorganic source of nitrogen. Heterotrophs get their nitrogen from amino acids and intermediate protein compounds such as peptones, peptides, proteases and peptides. Beef extract provides nitrogen needs for heterotrophs. Beef extract is rich in amino acids, vitamins, carbohydrates and mineral salts (phosphate and sulphate).

iv) **Minerals:** All organisms require several metallic elements such as sodium, potassium, calcium, magnesium, manganese, iron, zinc, copper, phosphorous and cobalt for normal growth.

v) **Growth Factors:** Any essential component of cell material that an organism is unable to synthesize from its basic carbon and nitrogen sources is classified as growth factors such as vitamins amino acids e.g. beef extracts, blood agar. Yeast extract provides vitamin B-complex.

vi) **Hydrogen Ion Concentration:** The growth of organisms in a particular medium may be completely inhibited if the pH of the medium is not within certain limits. The enzymes of microorganisms are greatly affected by this factor. Most bacteria grow best at around pH 7 or slightly lower. The pH of nutrient broth is adjusted to pH 6.8.

vii) **Agar:** Agar is used as solidifying agent because of its gel forming abilities and setting below 40°C and melting temperature of 90-95°C. Agar is derived from the polysaccharide agarose, which forms the supporting structure in the cell walls of certain species of algae. Agar is actually the resulting mixture of two components: the linear polysaccharide agarose, and a heterogeneous mixture of smaller molecules called agaropectin.

Agar is obtained from marine algae primarily from the genera *Gelidium* and *Gracilaria*. For commercial purposes, it is derived primarily from *Gelidium amansii*.

II. Different Types of Media

Different types of media used are classified as follows:

i) **Simple or basic Media:** The common example of simple or basic media is nutrient agar and nutrient broth. Nutrient agar is a solid medium which supports the growth of many microorganisms which do not have special nutrient requirements. It is used to maintain culture of bacteria.

ii) **Nutrient Media:** Nutrient media contain all the elements that most bacteria need for growth and are non-selective, so they are used for the general cultivation and maintenance of bacteria kept in laboratory culture collections. *Example*- Nutrient Agar

iii) **Minimal Media:** Minimal media are those that contain the minimum nutrients possible for colony growth, generally without the presence of amino acids, and are often used by microbiologists and geneticists to grow "wild type" microorganisms.

iv) **Enriched Media**: Enriched media contains additional substances which act as growth stimulants. For example, blood, serum, egg, vitamin etc. are used for enriching the media such as blood media, egg media etc. Enrichment Media it becomes easy to isolate a pathogen from specimen or mixed culture. This can be achieved by suppressing the undesirable organisms. For example selenite F broth is used as enrichment medium for isolation of Salmonella from stools prior to subculturing on Zylose Lysine Deoxycholate (XLD) agar.

v) **Selective Media:** Selective media are used for the growth of only selected microorganisms. It has presence or absence of specific components (like, presence of antibiotics, absence of any nutrient) to prevent the growth of microorganisms other than that of interest. *Example*- Eosine Methylene Blue media.

vi) **Differential Media:** Differential media or indicator media distinguish one microorganism type from another growing on the same media. This type of media uses the biochemical characteristics of a microorganism growing in the presence of specific nutrients or indicators (such as neutral red, phenol red, eosine or Methylene blue) added to the medium to visibly indicate the defining characteristics of a microorganism. *Example*- Blood Agar.

vii) **Indicator Media:** Indicator Media contains indicator which brings about colour change when bacterium grows in them e.g. Bismuth Sulphite Agar for *Salmonella typhii* which produces jet black colonies.

III. Preparation of Media

As per instructions media is diluted in distilled water. The liquid mixture is then subjected to autoclaving as per requirement.

13

Study of Different Basic Microbial Methods

Introduction

Microbiology techniques are used for various objectives like:

- To observe and isolate the micro-flora
- To test the microbiological quality of various food and dairy products
- To find the presence of any particular pathogenic microorganism
- To maintain a pure or mixed culture of specific microorganisms

1. Serial Dilution Techniques

- Bacteria are often present in such huge numbers that they can be difficult to count. Yet accurate counts are necessary for a variety of reasons like, for instance, assessing the quality of water or the safety of food. There are a number of counting techniques but most rely on the dilution of the sample to reduce the bacterial numbers down to a quantity that can be counted accurately.
- All bacterial plate count methods require the sample to be serially diluted until an estimated count of 30-300 colony forming units (CFU) on the plate is obtained. Plates with more than 300 CFU are very difficult to count. Plates with less than 30 CFU are not statistically reliable.
- If turbidity is observed in a broth culture, it might have millions more bacteria than you need. If this turbid broth is used directly for plating, all the CFU would grow together into a confluent mass and we would not be able to distinguish one colony from another.
- Traditionally serial dilutions were done with 1mL pipettes and 99ml sterile dilution bottles because they were the most accurate measuring devices available. With the advent of accurate and reliable micro-pipettors, smaller volumes can be used (0.1mL in 9.9ml or less of diluents). The important part of both methods is to ensure there is adequate mixing of your dilutions. Serial dilutions are generally made

in diluents like phosphate buffer, saline solution or sterile water. For ease of calculation, dilutions are done in multiples of 10 or 100.

- A single dilution is calculated as follows:

$$Dilution = \frac{Volume\ of\ sample}{Total\ volume\ of\ sample + Diluent\ volume}$$

- When doing very high dilutions (like 1/10,000 or 1/1,000,000), it is more accurate to do the dilution in a series of smaller dilutions rather than in one giant dilution. This is called a dilution series or a serial dilution.
- A typical dilution series is shown below

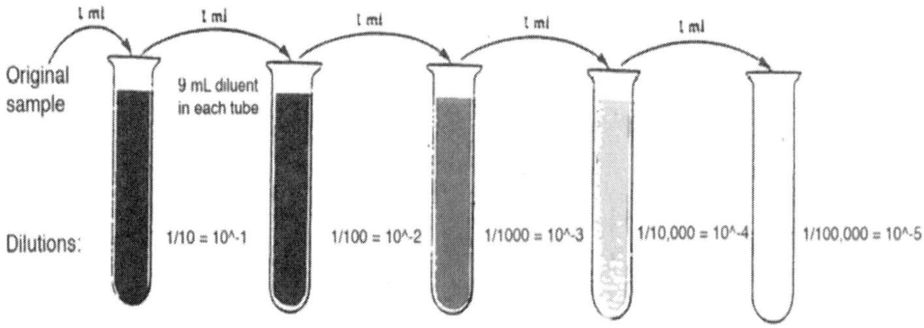

Fig. : Serial Dilution Technique

2. Plating Techniques

Sample, serial dilution or pure culture, are poured and spread on sterile solid media in petri-plates. The bacteria will grow into colonies, where it is assumed that one bacterium is enough to generate a full new colony of bacteria. That is termed as 1 **colony forming unit (cfu).**

Various plating techniques are described below:-

i) Pour Plating

- The pour plate technique can be used to determine the number of microbes/mL or microbes/gram in a specimen. It has the advantage of not requiring previously prepared plates, and is often used to assay bacterial contamination of food stuffs.
- The principle steps are :
  - Prepare/Dilute the sample
  - Place an aliquot of the diluted sample in an empty sterile plate
  - Pour 15ml of melted agar which is cooled to 45°C, swirl to mix

- Let it cool undisturbed to solidify on a flat table top
- Invert and incubate to develop colonies

- Each colony represents a "colony forming unit" (CFU). For optimum accuracy of a count, the preferred range for total CFU/plate is between 30 to 300 colonies/plate.
- One disadvantage of pour plates is that embedded colonies will be much smaller than those which happen to be on the surface, and must be carefully scored so that none are overlooked. Also, obligate aerobes may grow poorly if deeply imbedded in the agar.

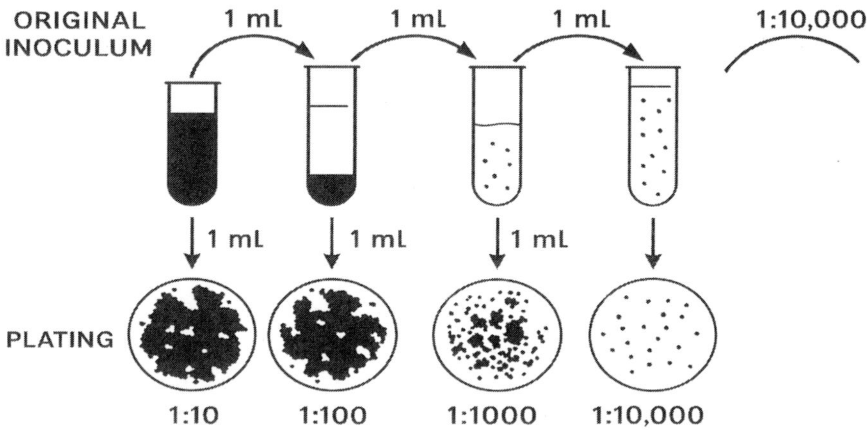

Fig. : Isolation of Pure Culture

ii) Spread Plating

- Another method of distributing bacteria evenly over the surface of an agar plate medium is commonly referred to as the spread plate method.
- A small volume of a bacterial suspension is spread evenly over the agar surface using a sterile bent glass rod as the spreading device. The goal in evenly distributing the bacterial suspension is typically to permit the growth of colonies that can subsequently be enumerated (see Serial Dilution Protocols) and/or sampled following incubation.
- Each plate is spread with single inoculums of the bacterial suspension.

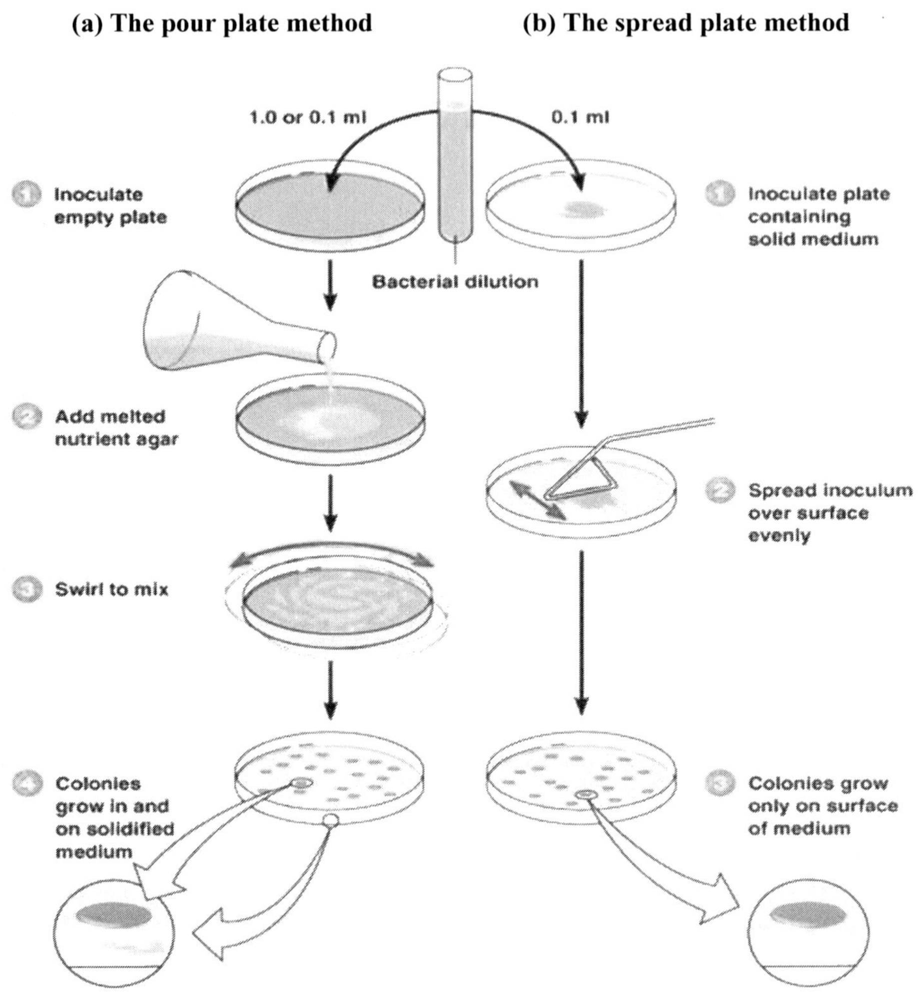

Fig. : Spread Plate Technique (Courtesy: www.canava.com)

iii) Drop Plate

- In drop plate method a fixed amount of microbiological sample (~20µl) is dropped directly on solid media surface under aseptic conditions.
- Each drop will spread and bacteria will form colonies.
- This method is faster and is usually used for enumeration of bacteria.

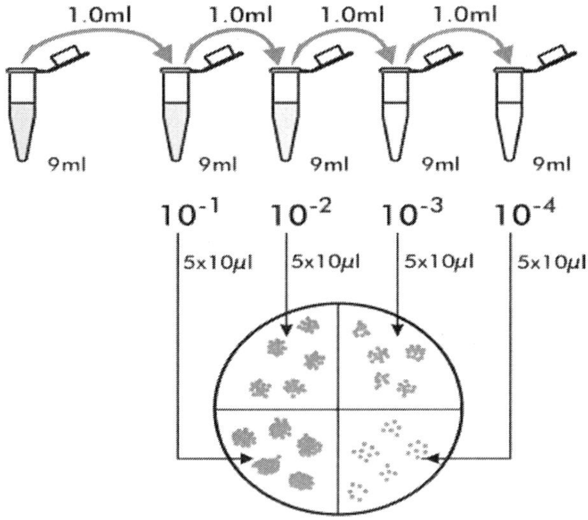

Fig. : Drop Plate Technique (Courtesy: www.canava.com)

iv) Streaking Method

- The streak plate method is a rapid qualitative isolation method.
- The techniques commonly used for isolation of discrete colonies initially require that the number of organisms in the inoculums be reduced. It is essentially a dilution technique that involves spreading a loopful of culture over the surface of an agar plate.

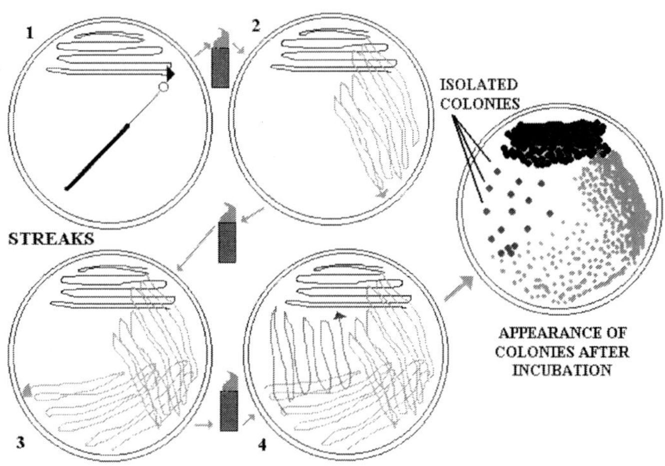

Fig. : Streak Plate Technique (Courtesy: www.canava.com)

- The resulting diminution of the population size ensures that, following inoculation, individual cells will be sufficiently far apart on the surface of the agar medium to effect a separation of the different species present.
- Although much type of procedures is performed, the four ways or quadrant streak is mostly done.

Questions

Why are agar plates incubated upside down? Two reasons :

1. Although there may be air contaminants in the incubator, it will be more difficult for them to get onto plates, and then move UP onto the agar to settle since gravity is working against this movement.
2. Often you will see a bit of water condensation on the petri dish cover. The water molecules are cohesive and tend to run together. If the plate is sitting right side up, the water droplets can fall onto the agar, creating a kind of little lake on the agar surface, messing up the plates. Upside down plates prevents the condensation from dropping on the agar surface.

14

Isolation Techniques for Pure Culture

Introduction

In order to study the cultural, morphological and physiological characteristics of an individual species, a pure culture of the microorganisms is required. Several different methods of separating the microorganisms from a mixed culture are available. The two most frequently used methods involve making a pour plate and/or streak plate. Isolated colonies are obtained from individual organisms after incubation.

Streak Plate Method

Plating is generally applied to the inoculation of a medium in petridish. Streak plate method is best for the separation of organisms from a mixed culture. In this method, agar medium is allowed to solidify as a thin layer in a petri dish and culture is streaked on the surface of agar medium and allowed to incubate to get isolated colonies.

Materials

1. Sterile petri plate
2. Wire loop
3. Nutrient agar medium
4. Bunsen burner
5. Mixed culture of *E.coli* and *Micrococcus leutus*

Procedure

1. Clean and disinfect the table top.
2. Liquefy the nutrient agar and cool to 50^0C.
3. Pour the medium into the bottom of the plate under aseptic conditions. Distribute the agar medium into the plate evenly.
4. Allow the agar to solidify. Dry the plates in the incubator at 37^0C for 1 day (hot medium will result in condensation of moisture on the cover which may drop down on the colonies and spread the colonies. Thus the isolation of microorganisms may be affected. Moisture on the surface of the medium may interfere with the production of discrete colonies).

5. Streak the plate by taking one loop full of mixed culture aseptically by continuous streaking or quadrant streaking method. Flame the loop every time. Apply the loop lightly. Don't gouge into the medium.
6. Flame the loop before placing it down.

Pour Plate Method

This method enables the number of living organisms or clump of organisms (i.e. colony forming units) in a sample to be counted, if subjected to appropriate medium and incubation conditions being used. In this method of separating one species of bacteria from another species, dilution of the known amount of sample in sterile diluents is done in such a manner that optimum number of organisms will be obtained in one of the plates poured.

Materials

1. Mixed culture of *E.coli*, *Bacillus subtilis*
2. Nutrient agar
3. Sterile petri plates
4. Dilution blank
5. Sterile pipettes
6. Marker

Procedure

1. Mix the sample thoroughly by shaking the tube or bottle 25 times or by inverting it 25 times.
2. Withdraw 1 ml of sample with 1 ml sterile pipette and transfer the contents to 9 ml saline tube carefully under aseptic conditions. Discard the pipette and label the first dilution tube.
3. Mix the contents of first dilution tube by shaking the tubes 25 times. Take up a fresh sterilized 1 ml pipette and withdraw 1 ml of the sample from 1st dilution and transfer it to second tube of 9 ml saline solution. Discard the pipette and label 2nd dilution on this tube.
4. Prepare 3rd, 4th and 5th, etc. dilutions in the same way using fresh sterile pipette every time.
5. Withdraw 1 ml of the contents of the last dilution and transfer the contents to a sterile petriplate. Touch the tip of the pipette against the dish to allow last drop to be transferred.
6. To each plate add molten agar medium at 45°C and immediately mix the medium and inoculums by circulating movement for 10-15 seconds. Avoid splashing of any medium into the lid or side of petri dish.

7. Allow the medium to solidify and incubate the plates inverted at 37ºC for 24 to 48 hours.
8. Select the plates showing colony forming units between 30 to 300 per plate.

Result & Interpretation

Questions

1. Which method requires more skill; streak plate or pour plate?
2. Why the Nutrient agar is cooled to 45^{0}C before incubating and pouring?
3. Why should a petri plate be discarded if media is splashed up the side or the top?
4. Why it is important to invert plates during incubation?
5. Why must loop be flamed before entering a culture?
6. Why must loop be flamed after making an inoculation?

15

Microbiology of Soil, Water, and Air

A. Enumeration of Different Microflora of Soil

Introduction

Agriculturally, soil is the region which supports the plant life by providing mechanical support and nutrients required for growth. From the microbiologist view point, soil is one of the most dynamic sites of biological interactions in the nature. Soil is an admixture of five major components viz. organic matter, mineral matter, soil-air, soil water and soil microorganisms/living organisms. The amount/ proposition of these components varies with locality and climate.

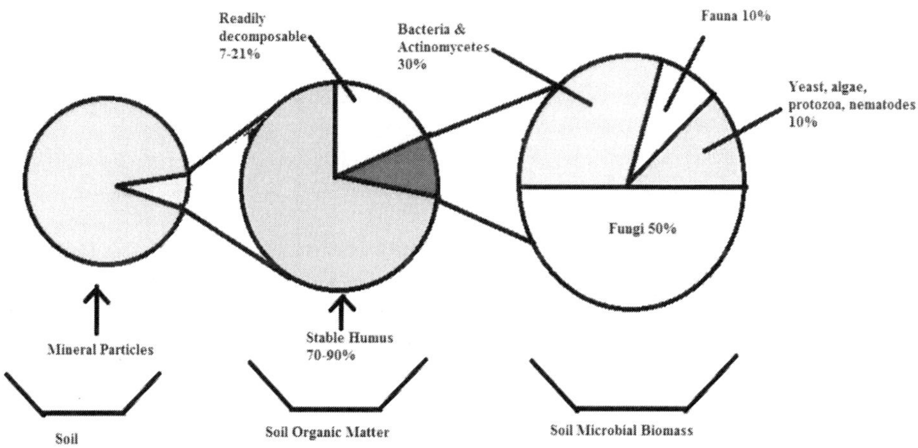

Fig. Major components of soil

The soil organisms are broadly classified in two group's viz. soil flora and soil fauna, the detailed classification of which is as follows.

1) Soil flora

a) Microflora Bacteria, Fungi, Molds, Yeast, Mushroom, Actinomycetes, Streptomyces, Algae e.g. BGA, Yellow Green algae, Golden brown algae.

b) Macroflora

1. Microfauna: Protozoa, Nematodes
2. Macrofauna: Earthworms, moles, ants and others. As soil inhabit several diverse groups of microorganisms, but the most important amongst them are: bacteria, actinomycetes, fungi, algae and protozoa.

Relative proportion/percentage of various soil microorganismsare: bacteria-aerobic (70%), anaerobic (13%), actinomycetes (13%), fungi/molds (3%) and others (algae, protozoa, viruses) 0.2-0.8 %. Number of organisms in a fertile agriculture soil per gram has been reported to contain 2.5 million bacteria, 0.45 million fungi and 0.7 million actinomycetes.

Materials

1. Sterile petridishes, spatula and pipettes
2. Nutrient agar tubes
3. Potato Dextrose Agar
4. Dilution blanks (99 ml and 9 ml)
5. Soil Samples

Procedure

1. Remove all the vegetation from the surface of farm soil.
2. Dig with a sterile spatula to a depth of 2-3 inch inside the soil.
3. Transfer about 20-25 grams of soil into a glass stoppered bottle.
4. Collect the samples from different places.
5. Add 11 gm. of soil to blank (99ml) shake vigorously for five minutes and make serial dilutions to 6th dilution using dilution blank tubes (9ml).
6. Transfer 1 ml of the suspension from 4, 5, 6 dilution to petriplate and pour melted and cooled nutrient agar for total bacterial counts.
7. Transfer 1 ml of dilution 1, 2, 3 to petriplate and add pour Potato Dextrose Agar (adjust pH of the medium using 10% sterile tartaric acid prior to pouring the agar. Add about 0.1 to 0.15 ml for 10 ml Potato Dextrose Agar)
8. Incubate all the plates at 30°C for 3-5 days.
9. Count the number of colonies in plates giving 30-300 colonies per plate.
10. Prepare smears of typical bacterial colonies in each plate at the end of incubation period and examine for morphology by Gram's staining.
11. Examine mold like colonies under low power objective of a microscope.

Observation

S. No.	Place of examination/ Source	Dilution	Total Count	Average count per gm	Types of organisms	Remarks
1. a. NA b. PDA						
2 a. NA b. PDA						
3 a. NA b. PDA						
4 a. NA b. PDA						

Result & Interpretation

Questions

1. Explain the role of microorganism in soil fertility?
2. Why are the plates incubated at 30°C and not at 37°C?
3. Why soil is considered as an excellent medium for microbial growth?
4. What is the microbial content in a fertile soil?
5. Do soil counts vary with depth? Why?

B. Enumeration of Different Microflora of Water Samples

Introduction

Water is essential to life. An adequate, safe and accessible supply must be available to all. Improving access to safe drinking water can result in significant benefits to health. According to the WHO, the mortality of water associated diseases exceeds 5 million people per year. From these, more than 50% are microbial intestinal infections, with cholera standing out in the first place. If water is polluted with faecal matter, sewage or manure, it is likely to contain many intestinal pathogens and communicate dangerous diseases like typhoid, cholera and dysentery to man. Natural water (e.g. streams, wells, tanks) may also be contaminated with a variety of microorganisms derived from soil vegetation and other sources. Mostly, Gram negative bacteria such as *Pseudomonas, Flavobacterium, Acinetobacter* and *Chromobacterium* and a few gram positive bacteria such as Micrococcus and Bacillus are present in water.

For assessing the sanitary quality of water it is generally examined for total bacterial content, for incidence of *Coliforms*, anaerobic sporeformers and fecal streptococci. Indicator organisms are bacteria such as non-specific *Coliforms, Escherichia coli* and *Pseudomonas aeruginosa* that are very commonly found in the human or animal gut and which, if detected, may suggest the presence of sewage or fecal water. Indicator organisms are used because even when a person is infected with more pathogenic bacteria, they will still be excreting many millions times more indicator organisms than pathogens. It is therefore reasonable to surmise that if indicator organism levels are low, then pathogen levels will be very much lower or absent.

A series of tests can be used to demonstrate the presence of *Coliform* sewage indicators in water supplies. A coliform is facultative anaerobes that ferment lactose to produce gas and is gram negative non-sporeforming rods e.g. *Escherichia coli* and *Enterobacter aerogenous*.

1. Estimation of Total number of Bacteria in Water (SPC)

Water organisms have great variability in physiological needs and no single medium, pH or temperature is ideal for all types. In spite of the fact that only small numbers of organisms in water will grow on nutrient media (due to the optimum temperature of it is 25°C) the standard plate count can perform an important function in water testing. Plate counts made of water before and after storage, can tell us how effective holding is in reducing bacterial numbers.

Much care is necessary in the collection of water samples for bacteriological analysis in order to secure truly representative samples from different sources of water and also to prevent any extraneous contamination of the samples at the time of collection. Samples containing less than 100 bacteria per ml are generally considered to be satisfactory and those having more than 1000 per ml as unsatisfactory.

Materials

1. Sample of Water
2. Tryptone Glucose Yeast Extract Agar(TGYA)

3. Dilution blanks(9 ml Saline)
4. Sterilized petriplates
5. Pipette 1 ml and 10 ml
6. Sample bottles
7. Ethyl Alcohol

Sampling of Tap Water

1. Allow the water to run for 3 or 4 minutes.
2. Clean the inside and outside of the nozzle of the top
3. Sterilize the nozzle of the tap by heating it with a blow lamp or a piece of ignited cotton-wool soaked in methylated spirit or Alcohol.
4. Again allow the tap to run slowly for about a minute.
5. Hold the sample bottle in one hand near the tap, remove the stopper with the other hand, flame the mouth of the bottle quickly bring the bottle below the running stream of water and when the bottle is nearly full, take it out and quickly replace the stopper.
6. The above operation must be carried out quickly to prevent undue exposure of the bottle to atmospheric contamination and to avoid any water failing on the outside of the mouth dripping inside.
7. Transport the bottle immediately to the laboratory and keep it in a refrigerator till required for analysis.

Sampling of Stream Water

1. If the water is shallow, care should be taken not to disturb the soil at the bottom.
2. Hold the bottle in one hand and gently lower it (with stopper on) into the stream as far below the surface as possible, remove the stopper with the other hand and as soon as bottle is full replace the stopper when the bottle is still under water and then take it out of the stream.
3. Take care to ensure that no floating or suspended materials fall into while taking the sample.
4. Wipe the exterior of the mouth and stopper with a clean cloth to prevent any water from dripping inside.
5. Transfer the sample to the laboratory at once for analysis.

Procedure

1. Shake water sample 25 times by moving up and down and prepare three water blanks with dilution of 1:10, 1:100 and 1:1000.

2. Pour 1ml of water sample from each of the dilution in petriplate in duplicate.
3. Pour melted and cool agar in each plate and mix thoroughly by rotating the plates.
4. Allow the agar to solidify and incubate one set of plates at 22°C for 72 hours and another at 37°C for 48 hours.
5. Select the pair of plates that has 30-300 colonies on each plate and count all the colonies on both plates.
6. Record the average count for the two plates on the laboratory report.

Observation

Sample	Source	Total viable count cfu/ ml At 37°C	Total viable count cfu/ml At 22°C	Remarks
1				
2				
3				
4				

Interpretation

Suggested standards for drinking water

Less than 100

TVC/ml	Remark
Less than 100	Satisfactory
More than 1000	Unsatisfactory

Calculation & Expression of Results

Case 1: Plates having microbial count between10 and 300 cfu

N = Colonies Plate1 + Colonies Plate 2

$$N = \frac{\text{Colonies Plate1} + \text{Colonies Plate 2}}{2}$$

Case 2: Plates having microbial countless than10cfu but at least 4.

Calculate the results as given in Case 1.

Case 3: If microbial load is from 3 to 1 then reporting of results shall be:

"Microorganisms are present, but, less than 4 per ml"

Case4: When the test sample/plates contain no colonies then reporting of results shall be:

"Less than 1 cfu/ml"

2. Detection of *E.coli* and Coliform

Coliform bacteria are a commonly used bacterial indicator of sanitary quality of foods and water. They are defined as rod-shaped Gram-negative non-spore forming and motile or non-motile bacteria which can ferment lactose with the production of acid and gas when incubated at 35–37°C. Typical genera include: *Citrobacter, Enterobacter, Hafnia, Klebsiella, and Escherichia.*

Coliforms can be found in the aquatic environment, in soil and on vegetation; they are universally present in large numbers in the feces of warm-blooded animals. While coliforms themselves are not normally causes of serious illness, they are easy to culture, and their presence is used to indicate that other pathogenic organisms of fecal origin may be present.

E.coli is Gram negative, facultative anaerobic, rod-shaped coliform bacteria, produce indole from tryptophan at 44 ± 0.5°C within 21 ± 3hr.

A. Principle

Lactose TTC Agar with Tergitol-7 is recommended as a selective and differential medium for the recovery of injured coliform organisms from water by membrane filtration technique. It also inhibits Gram positive bacteria. Lactose fermentation by Coliform results in development of yellow colonies, however lactose fermenting organism produce blue colonies.

B. Culture Media

- Lactose TTC agar with sodium heptadecyl sulphate (Tergitol-7Agar)
- Tryptophan broth
- Tryptone Soya agar (Soyabean Case in digest agar)

C. Procedure

- Disinfect the surface of the bottle/pouch/cups containing sample with 70% ethanol.
- Thoroughly mix the sample by vigorous shaking to achieve uniform distribution.
- Filter the sample (requisite volume) through a sterile membrane filter (0.45µm pore size) and place the filter on Lactose TTC agar plates. Incubate at 36 ± 2ºC for 21±3hr.
- Examine the membrane and count characteristic colonies of lactose-positive bacteria, showing yellow color development in the medium under the membrane.

- In case of not typical growth after 21 ± 3h, incubation may be further extended upto 44 ± 4hr at 36 ± 2°C.
- Examine the membrane for lactose positive colonies, irrespective of size showing yellow color development under the membrane.
- Further subculture the presumptive colonies on non-selective agar (Tryptone Soya Agar) and incubate at 36 ± 2°C for 21 ± 2 hr to carry out oxidase test.
- Also inoculate presumptive colonies in Tryptophane broth tube at 44 ± 0.5°C for 21 ± 3 hr and examine for indole production by adding Kovac's reagent for development of cherry-red colour at surface of the broth to confirm the production of indole.
- Consider all colonies giving negative oxidase reaction as Coliform.
- Consider all colonies giving negative oxidase reaction and positive indole reaction as *E.coli.*

Expression of Results

Presence/Absence of *E.coli* and Coliform given after confirmation of presumptive colonies in the sample examined.

Test for *E.coli* and Coliform=Present/absent per X ml of sample

3. Test for Coliform (MPN Method)

The Coliform group includes all the aerobic and facultative an aerobic gram negative, non-spore forming rod shaped bacteria which ferment lactose with gas formation within 48hr at 37°C.

Principle: Multiple tube dilution tests include presumptive, confirmed & completed tests as total independent procedures. The results are actually estimate based on certain probability formula. The most satisfactory information is obtained when the largest portion examined shows no gas in all or majority of the tubes. The most probable number (MPN) value for a given sample is obtained by the use of MPN tables.

Culture Media

- MacConkey broth
- Brilliant green bile lactose broth
- Nutrient agar
- MacConkey agar
- Lactose broth

Procedure

Presumptive Test

i. Inoculate a series of MacConkey broth tubes with appropriate measured quantities of water to be tested (50ml x1, 10 ml x5,1ml x5 and 0.1ml x 5).

ii. Inoculate all the tubes at 37°C for 24-48 hr.

iii. Examine each tube at the end of 24 ± 2 hr. for gas production and if no gas has been formed, re-incubate up to 48 hr.

iv. Record the presence or absence of the gas at each examination of the tube regardless of the amount.

v. The absence of gas formation at the end of 48 ± 3hour in any amount in inner fermentation tube constitutes a negative test.

Confirmed Test

i. Transfer a loopful of culture from positive tubes of MacConkey broth to Brilliant Green broth (BGB). During such transfer gently shake the tube or mix by rotating.

ii. Incubate the inoculated tubes at 37°C for 48 ± 3hr.

iii. The formation of gas in any amount in the Durahm tubes of BGB tubes at any time within 48 ± 3hr constitutes positive confirmed test.

Completed Test

i. Streak a loopful from positive BGB tube to MacConkey agar plates. Incubate at 37°C for 24 ± 2hr.

ii. From each plate pick typical colony and inoculate in Lactose broth and Nutrient agar slants. Incubate at 37°C for 24 to 48 hr.

iii. Pick up the strain from Nutrient agar and Gram stain. Coliform is gram negative, non-spore forming bacilli.

iv. Observe Lactose broth for gas formation after incubation. Coliform shows gas production.

Special Precautions

The concentration of nutritive ingredients in the mixture should be sufficient and as per requirements 0.1ml & above aliquots should be inoculated in double strength and 1ml and its dilutions should be inoculated in single strength medium.

4. Method for Detection of Yeast & Moulds

These are microbes which are capable of forming colonies in a selective medium (Chloramphenicol Glucose Yeast Extract Agar medium) at 25°C. Chloramphenicol Yeast Glucose Agar is a selective medium recommended for isolation and enumeration of Yeast & Moulds. The medium contains yeast extract, which provide nitrogenous nutrient and vitamin-B complex. Dextrose is the energy source. Chloramphenicol a thermo-stable antibiotic, suppresses the bacterial flora. Aerobic incubation of plates is done at 25°C ± 1°C and count is taken on 3rd, 4th or 5thday.

Culture media

Chloramphenicol Glucose Yeast Extract Agar (CGYEA)

Procedure

1. Aseptically clean the surface of bottle/pouch/cups containing sample with 70% ethanol and filter 250ml (or as specified) of water sample through a membrane filter of 0.45µm pore size using sterile membrane filtration assembly.
2. Place the filter on CGYEA media and incubate at 25 ± 1°C.

Observation

Observe the plates for colonies of Yeast & Moulds on 3rd, 4th and 5th days of incubation.

It is advisable to examine the plates at the end of three days for yeast colonies, which are smooth, moist, elevated or surface colonies. Mould colonies are easily recognized by the profuse growth of hyphae.

Expression of results

Presence/Absence of yeast & Moulds given after examining the plates of sample.

Test for Yeast and Moulds = Present/absent per X ml of sample

C. Enumeration of Different Microflora of Found in Air

Introduction

Air is not a natural environment for the growth and reproduction of microorganisms but a few types organisms (e.g. aerobic spore-formers, Micrococci, Mold spores) may, however, be found in association with dust particles suspended in the air. In the vicinity of cattle shed, dairies and fermentation industries, the atmosphere may carry several types of bacteria, yeasts, mold spores and bacteriophages. Air is also known to be a medium for the transmission of infectious microorganisms (e.g. viruses). The air inside a bacteriological laboratory is frequently required to be sterilized by irradiation of fumigation by bactericidal chemicals (aerosol).

A knowledge of the numbers and types of microorganisms present in the atmosphere inside dairies, cattle yards, food factories, is very important for controlling contamination of milk, milk products and other materials.

Materials

1. Sterile petri dishes
2. Nutrient agar tubes
3. Sabourauds agar tubes

Procedure

1. Pour two plates with melted nutrient agar and two plates with sabouraud's agar. Allow the media to set and harden.
2. Remove the tops of the plates. Expose the plates of each medium on the laboratory bench, garden and office for 15 minutes. Immediately replace the tops.
3. Incubate the nutrient agar plates at 30^0C for 48 hours and sabouraud's agar plates at 22^0C for 72 hours.
4. Count the number of colonies in each plate and examine for morphology by Gram's staining.
5. Prepare smears of typical bacterial colonies in each plate at the end of incubation period.
6. Examine mold like colonies under low power objective of a microscope.

Observation

S. No.	Place of examination/ Place of Air sampling	Time of exposure of agar plates	Total Count	Total count per cubic feet per minute	Types of organisms	Remarks
1. a. NA b. Sabouraud's Agar						
2 a. NA b. Sabouraud's Agar						

3 a. NA b. Sabouraud's Agar						
4 a. NA b. Sabouraud's Agar						

Interpretation

Number of organisms per cubic feet per minutes, should not exceed ONE for satisfactory atmosphere

Questions

1. Is air a good medium for growth of microorganisms?
2. What types of organisms are present in air?
3. Why pigmented organisms are present in air?
4. What is the microbial content in fresh air outside the city?
5. At what altitudes can you find microorganisms in air?

16

Enumeration of Microbial Growth

(A) Enumeration of Microbial Growth by Turbidity Measurement Method and Estimation of Generation Time

Introduction

Bacterial growth usually refers to reproduction-increase in population size-rather than to enlargement of mycelia cells. "Reproduction in bacteria occurs mainly through binary (binary means one cell becomes two) or transverse fission that results in the formation of two daughter cells. This is repeated at intervals by each new daughter cell in turn, or with each successive round of division. The population increases (Fig. 1). The time required for a complete fission cycle i.e. parent cell to two daughter cells is called the generation or doubling time. In bacteria, it is a doubling process in which each new fission cycle or generation increases the population by a factor of 2. So the parent stage consists of 2 cells, the second of 4, then 8, 16, 32, 64, 128, 256 and so on (Fig. 2). Thus the population will double, over and over again as long as the environment remains favorable for growth. The length of generation time is a measure of the growth rate of an organism. The average generation time in bacteria is 30-60 minutes under optimum conditions. Some species have very rapid growth rate and short generation time (5-10 minutes) and others have very slow growth rates and long generation times (measured in days). *Staphylococcus aureus* and *Salmonella enteritidis*, both causes of food poisoning, are examples of pathogens having relatively short doubling times of 20-30 minutes, which result in a few million cells from a few cells in a few hours in the infested food. The longest generation time occurs in species of Mycobacterium, particularly *Mycobacterium leprae* (the cause of leprosy) of 10-30 days as long as in some animals.

Determination of bacterial growth requires inoculation of a sterile broth medium and incubation of the culture under optimum temperature and gaseous conditions. The bacteria will reproduce rapidly under these conditions and the microbial growth may be measured by a variety of techniques, viz. dry weight determination, determination of total nitrogen by Kjeldahl method, direct

(Plate count) which detects living organisms by their ability to form colonies on agar surfaces, and turbidity measurements, which relate cell number to the turbidity (cloudiness) of a broth culture. Turbidity or optical density (OD) is not a direct measure of bacterial numbers, but increase in turbidity does indicate bacterial growth. OD is directly proportional to cell concentration.

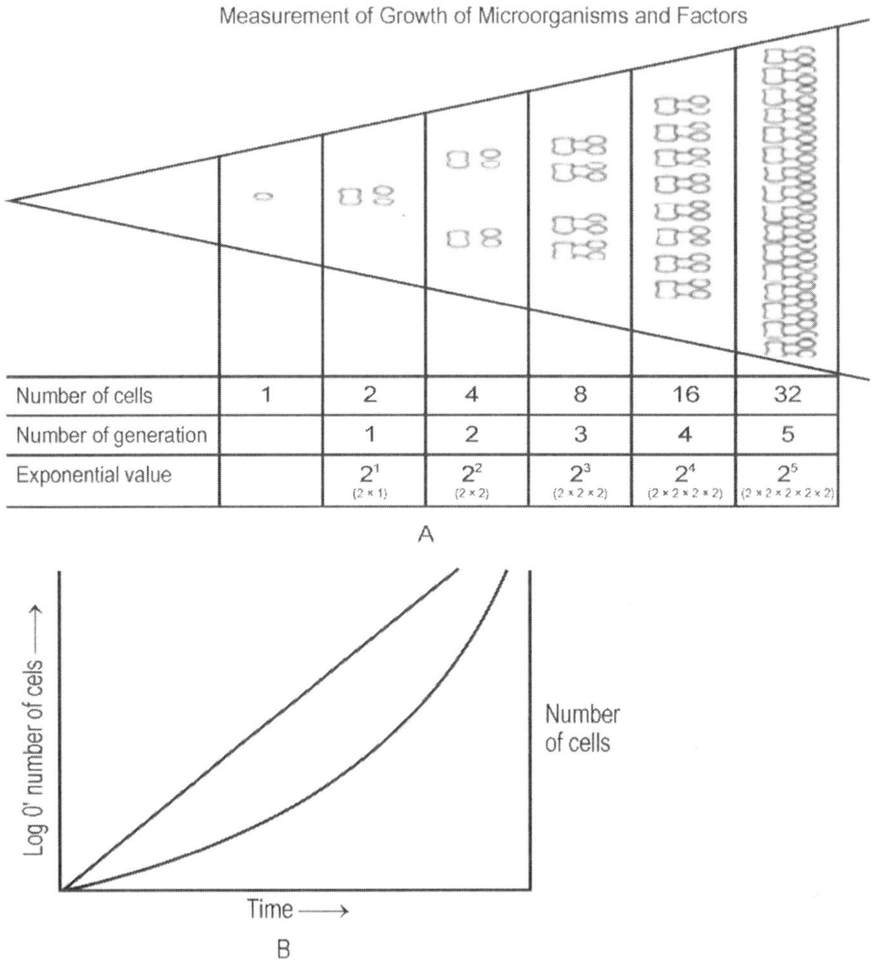

Fig. The mathematics of population grown, (A) Starting with a single cell, if each product of reproduction goes on to divide in a binary fashion, the population doubles with each new division cycle or generation. This procees can be represented by simple numbers of by logarithms (2 raised to an exponent). (B) Plotting the cell number arithmetically gives a curved slope. whereas plotting the logarithm of the cells production a straight line indicative of exponential growth.

In the laboratory, turbidity is measured with a photoelectric colorimeter (e.g. Bausch and Lomb Spectronic 20 and 21, Klett and summers on colorimeter or Zeiss Spekol spectrophotometer), and instrument that measures the amount of light transmitted directly through a sample. With the increase of bacterial numbers, the broth becomes, more turbid, causing the light to scatter and allowing less light to reach the photoelectric cell. The change in direction of light is indicated in the spectrophotometer as percentage or % T (the amount of light passing through the suspension) and absorbance (a value derived from the percentage of transmission).

Absorbance [(A = -log %T/100)] is a logarithmic value, more linear than %T and is used to plot bacterial growth curve on a graph. The relationship between % T and absorbance is exactly the same as the relationship between %T and OD. Thus you can read the values on the log scale (Abs) and consider these to be OD values. Bacterial growth curve construction requires that samples of a 24-hours shake-flask culture be measured for population sizes at regular time intervals during the incubation period. The bacterial growth curve (Fig.1) shows four distinct phases of growth, the lag phase, logarithmic phase, stationary phase and death phase, the actual length of each phase varies with the organisms and with environmental conditions.

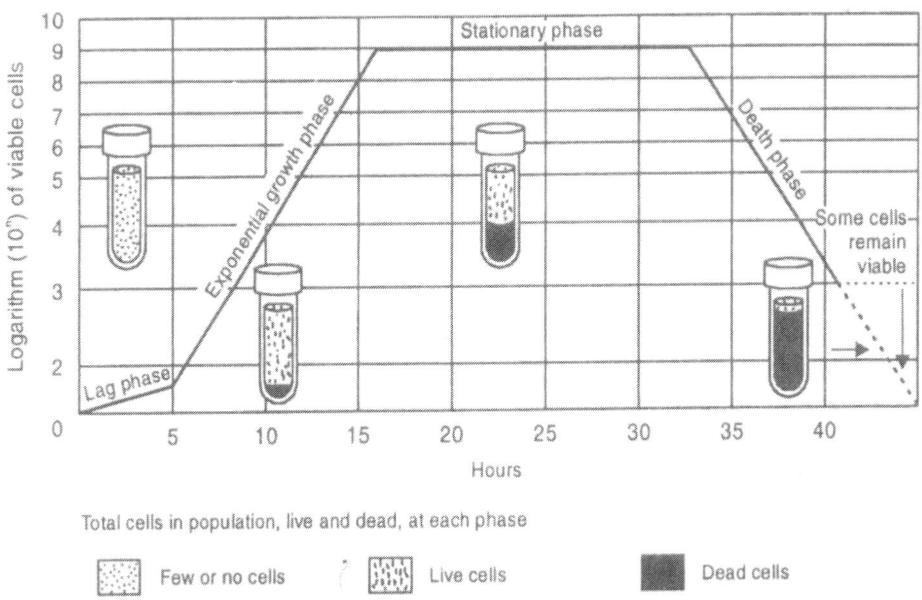

Fig. The bacterial growth curve showing the four typical phases of growth. On the graph the number of viable cells expressed as logarithm (log) is plotted against time. Cells are multiplying and dying all ao = long the curve, but the relative rates of these events change as the curve proceeds (modified from Talaro, K. and Talaro, A. (1996). Foundations in Microbiology. 2nd Ed. Wm.c. Brown Publishers, USA

Requirements

- 10-hour to 10-hour broth cultures of *Escherichia coli* (maintained at lag phase by immersion in an ice-water bath).
- Sterile 5-ml pipettes
- Brain-heart infusion broth (100 ml)
- Water Bath shaker incubator (at 37°C)
- Spectrophotometer
- 13 ×100 mm cuvettes
- Bunsen burner

Procedure

1. Aseptically transfer 5ml of the broth culture to 100 ml of brain-heart infusion broth flask.
2. Determine the initial OD (i.e. at To) at 600 nm wavelength which should be 0.08 to 0.01.
3. Place the inoculated culture flask in the shaker set at 120 rpm at 37°C for 6 hours.
4. Aseptically transfer after 30 minutes incubation, 5 ml of the culture to a cuvette.
5. Determine the optical density of the sample at 600 nm.
6. Repeat the steps 4 and 5 at each 30-minutes interval for a period of 6 hours.

Observations and Results

Record optical densities of the broth culture suspension at 30-minute time intervals for 6 hours in a tabular form as follows.

Culture (minutes of incubation)	Optical* density @ 600nm
0	
30	
60	
90	
120	
150	
180	
210	
360	

*Optical density (OD= .2-log of per cent transmittance).

Examples

If the percent transmittance of one of your sample is 53.5, solve the problem in the following way:

OD = 2-log of 53.5

= 2-1.7284 (.7284 is the value found in the log table is the mantissa.)

= 272

Plot a graph between optical versus incubation time, to prepare the growth curve and calculate the generation for the *E.coli* culture.

(B) Microbial Growth Measurement by Total Plate Count Method:

Introduction

The standard plate count is widely employed to determine the number of variable organisms in the sample of milk and other food items. The technique normally performed accounts for the number of viable aerobic and facultative anaerobic, mesophilic bacteria in the samples tested.

A small quantity of the sample mixed with nutrient agar in a Petri plates are incubated at a specified temperature for a definite period of time.

Each colony is presumed to have grown from one bacterium or clump of bacterial cell present in the inoculums. The total number of colonies counted on the plates multiplied by the dilution factor is taken to represent number of viable organisms in the sample.

Plate count methods determine the quantity of anaerobic and facultative aerobic, mesophilic bacteria per unit volume of food sample tested. The standard plate count method is the fundamental procedure from which other plate count methods have been derived. With minor modifications such as employing various agar media, changing incubation temperatures, and holding times, other plate count methods for the enumeration of special groups of microbes such as proteolytic types, lipolytic types, psychrophilic counts, thermoduric counts, thermophilic counts, coliform counts, etc. may be derived.

Materials

1. Incubator (37°C)
2. Bacteriological pipettes (1.1 ml)
3. Dilution blanks (9 ml, 99 ml)
4. Standard petri-plates (outside diameter- 97.8mm, inside diameter- 94mm and depth- 15mm)
5. Tryptone glucose yeast extract agar
6. Samples

Procedure

A. Mixing the sample and preparation of dilution

1. Mix the liquid sample by inverting the bottle about 6 times.
2. Remove 11 ml of the sample using a sterile bacteriological pipette and transfer it to the first tube of 99 ml diluents.
3. Allow the sample to drain out of the pipette and gently blow out the last drop.
4. Mix the contents completely by rotating the tubes between palms of the hand or use vortex mixer. This makes a dilution (1:10) into 9 ml. dilution blank to get 1:100 dilution (first).
5. Transfer 1 ml of first dilution (1:10) into 9ml dilution blank to get 1:100 dilution (second).
6. Similarly prepare a series of dilution as required, Use fresh pipette each successive dilution.

B. Preparation and incubation of plates

1. Using a fresh pipette transfer 1 ml of each required dilution into sterile petri dishes in duplicate.
2. Allow the contents to drain, touch the tip of the pipette to a dry place in the petri dish to drain out the last drop.
3. Add 15-18 ml Tryptone Glucose Yeast Extract agar previously melted and cooled to 42°C to 45°C into the sterile petri plates.
4. Mix the contents of the plates thoroughly by gently rotating the petri plate and allow the agar to cool and set.
5. Invert the plates and incubate at 37°C for 48 hours.

C. Counting the Colonies

1. Remove the plates from incubator after 48 hours and select the plates having colonies ranging 30 to 300 on each plate. (Note: plates having colonies between 25 to 250 on each plates are followed in some laboratories.)
2. Count the colonies with the aid of colony counter, find out the average number of counts and multiply these counts by the dilution factor.
3. Express the results as standard plate count for one milliliter of sample.
4. Enter the readings in the following table.

Sample	Dilution	Counts in plates		Average	SPC/ml	Inference
		1	2			

Interpretation

Questions

1. What are the limitations of the standard plate count?
2. Why area the petri dishes inverted during the incubation period?
3. Why area the plates incubated at 37°C?
4. List the sources of error in this method.
5. Why is the milk samples diluted for plate count procedures?
6. Why the 12-15 ml agar is medium recommended for each agar plate?
7. Define dilution factor.
8. Does the SPC method reveal the true total count of the milk sample? why ?
9. Why is a duplicate plate used?

17

Study the Effect of Different Physiological Factors on the Growth of Microbes

(A) Effect of Temperature

Introduction

Temperature is one of the most important physical factors affecting micro-organisms. Bacteria are different from higher plants and animals in the lack of homeostatic mechanism and cannot regulate heat generated by metabolism and are, therefore, directly and readily affected by temperature. Over a limited temperature range, there is a two-fold increase in the rate of enzyme catalyzed reaction for every 10°C rise in temperature.

Bacteria may be divided into three major groups with respect to their temperature requirements: (i) Psychrophiles, those with optimum temperature between 0°C and 20°C; (ii) Mesophiles, with optimum temperature between 20ºC and 40°C and (iii) Thermophiles, with optimum temperature between 40°C and 80°C. Thermophiles are of two types: (a) Facultative thermophiles with an optimum temperature of growth between 45°C and 60°C and (b) Obligate thermophiles with optimum temperature above 60°C. Temperatures in the range between 50°C and 100°C are normally in the lethal range for bacterial cells and spores. The range of temperature preferred by bacteria is genetically determined, resulting in enzymes with different temperature requirements.

Each organism grows within a particular temperature range (i.e. cardinal temperature points). The minimum growth temperature is the lowest temperature at which growth of a species will occur. The highest temperature at which a species can grow is its maximum growth temperature, and a species grows fastest at its optimum growth temperature.

Time of exposure is a vital factor in assessing the lethal effect of high temperature on bacterial cells. For this purpose two methods are useful; (i) the thermal death point (TDP), the temperature at which an organism is killed in 10 minutes of exposure; and (ii) thermal death time (TDT), is the time required to kill/spores suspension at a given temperature.

Effect of incubation temperature on growth :

Requirements

- Cultures of *Alternaria alternata, Chartomium thermophile* (fungi), *E.coli, Bacillus globisporus* and *Bacillus stearothermophilus.*
- Nutrient agar slants (18)
- Czapek-Dox agar plates (12)
- Bunsen burner
- Inoculating loop
- Inoculating needle
- Refrigerator set at 4°C
- Four incubators set at 15°C, 35°C, 55°C, and 75°C.

Procedure

1. Label each of the nutrient agar slants with the test organisms and the temperature of incubation (0, 4, 15, 35, 55, 75°C)
2. Inoculate six nutrient agar slants (labeled 0, 4, 15, 35, 55, 75°C) with *E.coli* by streaking the surface of each slope.
3. Repeat step 2 for inoculation of the remaining cultures.
4. Label each of the Czapek-Dox agar plates with *A. alternate* and *C. thermophile* and the temperature of incubation (0,5,15,35,55,75°C)
5. Inoculate six Czapek-Dox agar plates with *A. alternate* and other six plates *with C. thermophile* by transferring a disc on the center of each plate.
6. Incubate one inoculates slant and plate from each set at 0°C (ice box of refrigerator), 4°C (refrigerator) for 10-14 days and other slants and plates at 15, 35, 55 and 75°C (incubators set at these temperatures) for 24-48 hours (bacterial) and 7-14 days (fungal cultures).

Observation & Results

Examine the cultures after two days incubation (incubated at 15, 35, 55 and 75°C) after 10-14 days incubation (at 0 and 4) for the presence (+) or absence (-) of growth and the degree of growth (i.e. minimal growth (+), moderate growth (2+), heavy growth (3+), very (maximum) growth (4+). Express the results in the form of a table and determine the minimum, maximum and optimum temperature ranges for each microorganism and classify each organism as psychrophile, mesophile thermophile.

Table : Growth observed in four test organism at various incubation temperatures

Species	*Amount of growth at (°C)						Cardinal temperature for each organism Minimum Maximum Optimum	Temperature classification (Thermophile, mesophile or psychrophile)
	0	4	15	35	55	75		
Alternaria alternate								
Chaetomiu-mthermophile								
E.coli								
Bacillus globispprus								
Bacillus stearothermophilus								

*Amount of growth to be indiacted as -, +, 2+, 3+, or 4+.

Conclusion

Bacillus globisporus is a psychrophile;

E.coli, Alternaria alternate, mesophiles and

Bacillus stearothermophilus, Chaetomium thermophile are thermophiles.

Precautions

Cultures incubated at higher temperature (55°C, 75°C) should be kept in moist chambers to avoid drying of the media.

B) Effect of pH

Introduction

The pH is the symbol for the logarithm of the reciprocal of hydrogen ion concentration (log/H^+) in gram atoms per liter (i.e. (power) of $(H^+)_{10)}$.

For example, a pH 4 indicates a concentration of 0.0001 or 10^{-4} gram atoms of hydrogen ions in one litre of solution. In other words, pH value is the negative exponent of the H^+ concentration. The measure of the relative acidity or alkalinity of a solution is called pH. pH is expressed as a number from 0 to 14. A more acidic solution at 0.01 (10^{-2}) M has a lower pH value (pH=2). p^H changes of the environmental has a profound influence on the growth, activities and survival of the microorganisms, each enzyme system of an organism has a particular pH range in which it can function. Like cardinal temperature points, an organism has maximum pH (i.e. the concentration of H^+ (alkali) below which an organism fails to grow), optimum pH (i.e. the concentration of H^+ where growth of an organism is maximum) and minimum pH (i.e. the concentration of H^+ (acid) above which a microorganism fails to grow). In other words, the pH values above and below which an organism fails to grow are respectively termed as the minimum and maximum hydrogen ion concentrations. Enzymes differ greatly in their pH optima.

Each species has the ability to grow within a specific pH range, which may be broad or limited, with the most rapid growth occurring within a narrow optimum range. Although specific pH range for bacteria is between 4 and 9, the optimum growth usually occurs between 6.5 and 7.5. But there are some notable exceptions, including the acetic acid bacteria and *Thiobacillus thioxidans* which grow in acidic pH below 4. For example *T. thioxidans* tolerate normal acid, i.e. pH 0. Therefore, organic acid, are used to preserve food like fermented dairy products. Fungi are usually more tolerant of higher acid condition than bacteria, with optimum activities at a pH of 4 to 6. These specific pH need reflect the organism's adaptation to their natural environment. This property is used in selective media for the growth of fungi and bacteria.

Many bacteria produce organic acids from carbohydrate degradation and alkali from protein breakdown and these may inhibit growth due to shifts in pH. Buffers are frequently added to culture media to neutralize these acids and alkali and to maintain equilibrium. Peptones, proteins and amino acids, because of their amphoteric nature, in complex media act as natural buffers. Phosphate salts are often using in chemically defined media as buffers.

This exercise deals with testing the degree of inhibition of microorganisms that results from media containing different concentrations of hydrogen ions.

Requirements

- Cultures of *E.coli*, *Staphylococcus aureus* (Bacteria), *Penicillium* sp. and *Saccharomyces cerevisiae* (fungi)
- Tubes containing sterile, buffered nutrient broth adjusted to pH 2.5, 3.5, 4.5, 5.5, 6.5, 7.5, 8.5 and 9.5 (4 each pH, i.e. total 32 tubes)
- Bunsen burner
- Sterile 10-ml pipettes.

Procedure

1. Label each of the nutrient broth tubes with pH of the medium (i.e. 2.5,3.5.........) and name of the organism to be inoculated.
2. Inoculated each of a series of the tubes (pH 2.5, 3.5, 4.5, 5.5, 6.5, 7.5, 8.5, 9.5) with *E.coli* by adding 0.1 ml of the culture to each tube.

3. Repeat step 2 for the inoculation of *S. aureus, Penicillium* and *S. cerevisiae* to various labeled tubes.
4. Incubate the bacterial inoculated tubes for 24-48 hours at 35ºC and fungal inoculated tubes for 72-120 hours at 25°C.

Observation & Results

Record the growth of each organism by using the symbols: (-) no growth; (+) slight growth; (++) moderate growth; (+++) best growth. Form the results, state the optimum pH, minimum pH and maximum pH for each microorganism.

Table: Growth observed in four test organism at various incubation temperatures

Species	***Amount of growth at (pH)**								**Cardinal pH for each organism Minimum Maximum Optimum**
	2.5	**3.5**	**4.5**	**5.5**	**6.5**	**7.5**	**8.5**	**9.5**	
E.coli									
Staphylococcus aureus									
Penicillium sp.									
Saccharomyces cerevisiae									

*Amount of growth to be indicated as -,+,2+,3+, or 4+.

Conclusion

18

Study of Growth Characteristics of Fungi

Introduction

A) Cultivation of Fungi

A **fungus** is any member of the group of eukaryotic organisms that includes microorganisms such as yeasts and molds, as well as the more familiar mushrooms. These organisms are classified as a kingdom, Fungi, which is separate from the other eukaryotic life kingdoms of plants and animals.

A characteristic that places fungi in a different kingdom from plants, bacteria, and some protests is chitin in their cell walls. Similar to animals, fungi are heterotrophy; they acquire their food by absorbing dissolved molecules, typically by secreting digestive enzymes into their environment. Fungi do not photosynthesize. Growth is their means of mobility, except for spores (a few of which are flagellated), which may travel through the air or water. Fungi are the principal decomposers in ecological systems. These and other differences place fungi in a single group of related organisms, named the *Eumycota* (*true fungi* or *Eumycetes*), which share a common ancestor (form a *monophyleticgroup*), an interpretation that is also strongly supported by molecular phylogenetics. This fungal group is distinct from the structurally similar myxomycetes (slime molds) and oomycetes (water molds). The discipline of biology devoted to the study of fungi is known as mycology. In the past, mycology was regarded as a branch of botany, although now known fungi are genetically more closely related to animals than to plants.

Fungi can be cultivated by using various agar media like PDA & Chloroamphenicol Glucose Yeast Extract Agar etc. Fungi are capable of forming colonies in a selective medium Chloroamphenicol Glucose Yeast Extract Agar medium at 25°C. Chloramphenicol Yeast Glucose Agar is a selective medium recommended for isolation and enumeration of Yeast & Moulds. The medium contains yeast extract, which provides nitrogenous nutrient and vitamin-B complex. Dextrose is the energy source. Chloramphenicol at her most able antibiotic, suppresses the bacterial flora. Aerobic incubation of plates is done at 25°C ± 1°C and count is taken on 3rd, 4th or 5thday.

Requirements

Culture media: Chloroamphenicol Glucose Yeast Extract Agar (CGYEA)

Procedure

1. Aseptically clean the surface of bottle/pouch/cups containing sample with 70% ethanol and filter 250 ml (or as specified) of water sample through a membrane filter of 0.45 μm pore size using sterile membrane filtration assembly.
2. Place the filter on CGYEA media and incubate at 25±1°C

Observation

Observe the plates for colonies of Yeast & Moulds on 3rd, 4th or 5th day of incubation. It is advisable to examine the plates at the end of three days for yeast colonies, which are smooth, moist, elevated or surface colonies. Mold colonies are easily recognized by the profuse growth of hyphae.

Expression of Results

Presence/Absence of Yeast & Moulds given after examining the plates of sample Test for Yeast and Moulds = Present/Absent per × ml of sample

Observation Table

S. No.	Sample	Dilution No.	Colony Counts		Average Count (Cfu/ml)
			Plate No. 1	Plate No.2 (Duplicate)	
1					
2					
3					

Results & Interpretation

B) Morphological Characteristics of Fungi

Microscopic examination of Yeasts

Introduction

Yeasts are single cell organisms larger than bacteria and belong to the group of fungi. They reproduce by budding. A bud or blastospore, forms as an outpoching of the parent cell. Bud may separate from the original cell or remain attached. In some yeasts, buds may remain attached to each other to form a pseudo-hyphae. Yeast also reproduces by formation of spores. Yeasts are commonly found in soil, fruits, food materials including dairy products like butter and cheese. They ferment sugars producing alcohol and carbon dioxide and are important in the brewery and baking industries.

Materials

1. Broth culture of Saccharomyces cerevesiae, *Kluveromyces lactis* and *Candida pseudotropicalis or* steak sample from above grown plates in Exercise A.
2. Methylene blue (0.1% aqueous)
3. Microscopic slides
4. Cavity slide
5. Coverslip

Procedure

1. Prepare hanging drop slide of the three cultures and a sample from above plates. Compare their morphological characteristics as observed under the oil-immersion objectives.
2. Prepare the slides of above samples by simple staining technique using methylene blue stain.
3. Observe the morphology of all the yeasts under oil immersion objective.
4. Draw the microorganisms showing the presence of buds and pseudo-hyphae, if present.

Observation

S. No.	Cultures	Shape	Budding	Pseudo-hyphae	Remarks
1.	*S.cerevisiae*				
2.	*K.lactis*				
3.	*C.pseudotropicalis*				
4.	Sample from plate				

Interpretation

Microscopic Examination of Molds

Molds are saprophytic or parasitic fungi commonly found in soil, water, stools and other environment. They occur in filamentous form and much larger than bacteria. The filaments of Molds are called hyphae which may be septate or aseptate. A mass of intermeshed hyphae as seen microscopically is a mycelium. Molds reproduce by both asexual and sexual means, Mold form characteristic "cottony" colonies on agar medium. Mold colonies differ in color from each other. The identification of Molds is based on surface, back side color, hyphae structure and types of spores.

Materials

1. Mold culture on Sabouraud's agar
2. Microscopic slides
3. Cover glass
4. Lacto phenol cotton blue stain
5. Dissecting needles

Procedure

1. Place the uncovered plate on the stage of microscope and examine the edge of a colored colony with the low power objective. Look for hyphal structure and spore arrangement. The white colonies generally lack spores and are difficult to identify.
2. Compare the colony characteristics and spores with the figures given in textbooks.
3. Make a wet mount slide by transferring a small amount of the culture with a dissecting needle to a drop of Lacto phenol cotton blue stain on a slide. Cover with the cover glass and examine under low power and high dry objectives. Refer again the figures given in textbooks.
4. Repeat the procedure in different colonies.

Observations

S. No.	Cultures	Hyphae	Asexual	Spores	Microscopic appearance	Remarks
1.						
2.						
3.						
4.						

Interpretation

Questions

1. What is mycelium?
2. What is hypha?
3. How are true yeasts differentiated from false yeasts?
4. What kind of asexual spores are seen in penicillium?
5. What type of hyphae is seen in Mucor and Rhizopus?
6. What kind of asexual spores are seen in Mucor and Rhizopus?

Appendices

Appendix-I: Equipment, Materials & Glassware

List of equipment/lab-wares required for microbiological analysis is given below-

1. Biosafety Cabinet/ Laminar Air Flow Chambers
2. Membrane Filtration assembly/apparatus with Membrane Filters with pore size 0.45 μm
3. BOD Incubators/Universal Incubator(s)
4. Autoclave(s)
5. Weighing Balance (s)
6. pH Meter(s)
7. Hot Plate/Heating Mantle(s)
8. Water bath(s)
9. Drying Oven (Hot air Oven(s)
10. UV Cabinet
11. Colony Counter
12. Microscope(s)
13. Vacuum pump(s)
14. Petri plates
15. Inoculation Loop of 3mm diameter
16. Inoculating Loop(s)
17. Anaerobic jar(s)
18. Auto pipettes (100-1000 μl,1-10ml)
19. Durhum tubes.
20. Forceps

Appendix-II: Composition of Media & Broth

Asparagine Proline Broth

Ingredients g/l	**strength Concentrated**	**Single**	
L-Asparagines	:	2.0	3.2
L-Proline	:	1.0	1.6
Dipotassium phosphate	:	1.0	1.6
Magnesium sulphate	:	0.5	0.8
Potassium sulphate	:	10.0	16.0
Final pH (at 25°C) 7.2±0.2			

Directions

Suspend above ingredients in 1000 ml distilled water containing 25 ml or 40 ml ethanol respectively. Heat to boiling to dissolve the medium completely. Distribute as desired in screw-capped bottles. Close the caps so that the seal in the lid just touches the tip of the bottle. Adjust the pH and sterilize by autoclaving at 15lbs pressure (121°C) for 15 minutes. Tighten the caps of the bottles immediately after removal from the autoclave to prevent loss of ethanol by evaporation. It is not advisable to use polypropylene caps without seals. Alternatively, ethanol may best sterilize separately by filtration and then added aseptically to the sterile cooled medium.

Baird Parker Agar Base

Ingredients	**g/l**
Casein enzymic hydrolysate	10.0
Meat extract	5.0
Yeast extract	1.0
Glycine	12.0
Sodium pyruvate	12.0
Lithium chloride	5.0
Agar	20.0
Final pH (at 25°C) 7.0±0.2	

Directions

Suspend above ingredients in 950 ml distilled water. Heat to boiling to dissolve the medium completely. Adjust the pH and sterilize by autoclaving at 15 lbs pressure (121°C) for 15 minutes. Cool to 50°C and aseptically adds 50 ml concentrated Egg Yolk Telluride Emulsion (commercially available). Mix well and pour into sterile Petri plates.

MacConkey Broth /Neutral Red

Ingredients	g/l
Peptic digest of animal tissue	20.0
Lactose	10.0
Bile Salts	5.0
Sodium Chloride	5.0
Neutral Red	0.075
Final pH (at 25°C) 7.4 ± 0.2	

Directions

Suspend above ingredients in 1000ml distilled water. Heat if necessary to dissolve the medium completely. Adjust the pH and distribute into tubes with inverted Durham's tubes. Sterilize by autoclaving at 15lbs pressure (121°C) for 15 minutes. Cool the tubes before inoculation.

Buffered Peptone Water

Ingredients	g/l
Casein enzymic hydrolysate	10.0
Sodium chloride	5.0
Disodium hydrogen phosphate, $12H_2O$	9.0
Mono potassium hydrogen phosphate	1.5
Final pH (at 25°C) 7.1 ± 0.1	

Directions

Suspend above ingredients in1000 ml distilled water. Heat if necessary to dissolve the medium completely. Adjust the pH and dispense as desired and sterilize by autoclaving at 15lbs pressure (121°C) for 15 minutes.

Chloramphenicol Yeast Glucose Agar

Ingredients	g/l
Yeast extract	5.0
Dextrose	20.0
Chloramphenicol	0.1
Agar	15.0
Final pH (at 25°C) 6.6±0.2	

Directions

Suspend above ingredients in 1000 ml distilled water. Heat to boiling to dissolve the medium completely. Adjust the pH and sterilize by autoclaving at 15lbs pressure (121°C) for 15 minutes. Mix well and pour into sterile Petri plates.

Lactose Broth

Ingredients	g/l
Peptic digest of animal tissue	5.0
Beef extract	3.0
Lactose	5.0
Final pH (at 25°C) 6.9 ± 0.2	

Directions

Suspend above ingredients in 1000 ml distilled water. Heat if necessary to dissolve the medium completely. Adjust the pH and distribute into tubes with inverted Durham's tubes. Sterilize by autoclaving at 15 lbs pressure (121°C) for 15 minutes. Cool the tubes before inoculation.

Mac Conkey Agar

Ingredients	g/l
Peptic digest of animal tissue	20.0
Lactose	10.0
Bile salts	5.0
Sodium chloride	5.0
Neutral red	0.07
Agar	15.0
Final pH (at 25°C) 7.5 ± 0.2	

Directions

Suspend above ingredients in1000 ml distilled water. Heat to boiling with gentle swirling to dissolve the medium completely. Adjust the pH and sterilize by autoclaving at 15lbs pressure (121°C) for 15 minutes. Avoid overheating. Cool to 45-50°C and pour into sterile Petri plates. The surface of the medium should be dry when inoculated.

Nutrient Agar

Ingredients	g/l
Glucose	1.0
Peptic digest of animal tissue	5.0
Beef extract	3.0
Agar	15.0
Final pH (at 25°C) 7.2 ± 0.2	

Directions

Suspend above ingredients in 1000 ml distilled water. Heat to boiling to dissolve the medium completely. Adjust the pH and sterilize by autoclaving at 15lbs pressure (121°C) for 15 minutes.

Overlay Agar Medium

Ingredients	g/l
Agar	12-18g
Water	1000ml
Final pH (at 25°C) 7.0 ± 0.2	

Directions

Suspend above ingredients in1000 ml distilled water. Heat if necessary to dissolve the medium completely. Adjust the pH and sterilize by autoclaving at 15lbs pressure (121°C) for 15 minutes.

Peptone Water

Ingredients	g/l
Peptic digest of animal tissue	20.0
Sodium chloride	5.0
Final pH (at 25°C) 7.4 ± 0.2	

Directions

Suspend above ingredients in 1000 ml distilled water. Heat if necessary to dissolve the medium completely. Adjust the pH and dispense in test tubes. Sterilize by autoclaving at 15lbs pressure (121°C) for 15 minutes.

Plate Count Agar (Standard Methods Agar)

Ingredients	g/l
Casein enzymic hydrolysate	5.0
Yeast extract	2.5
Dextrose	1.0
Agar	15.0
Final pH (at 25°C) 7.0 ± 0.2	

Directions

Suspend above ingredients in 1000ml distilled water. Heat if necessary to dissolve the medium completely. Adjust the pH and dispense in test tubes. Sterilize by autoclaving at 15lbs pressure (121°C) for 15 minutes. Mix well and pour into sterile Petri plates.

Tergitol-7 Agar Base

Ingredients	g/l
Peptic digest of animal tissue	10.0
Yeast extract	6.0
Meat extract	5.0
Lactose	20.0
Sodium heptadecyl sulphate (Tergitol 7)	0.10
Bromothymol blue	0.05
Agar	16.0
Final pH (at 25°C) 7.2±0.1	

Directions

Suspend above ingredients in 1000 ml distilled water. Heat if necessary to dissolve the medium completely. Adjust the pH and sterilize by autoclaving at 15lbs pressure (121°C) for15 minutes. Cool to 45-50°C. Add 5ml of 0.05% of Triphenyl Tetrazolium Chloride (TTC). Mix well and pour into sterile Petri plates.

Triple Sugar Iron Agar

Ingredients	g/l
Peptic digest of animal tissue	20.0
Meat extract	3.0
Yeast extract	3.0
Lactose	10.0
Sucrose	10.0
Glucose	1.0
Ferric citrate	0.3
Sodium chloride	5.0
Sodium thiosulphate, pentahydrate	0.3
Phenol red	0.024
Agar	12.0
Final pH (at 25°C) 7.4 ± 0.2	

Directions

Suspend above ingredients in 1000ml distilled water. Heat if necessary to dissolve the medium completely. Adjust the pH and distribute into test tubes. Sterilize by autoclaving at 15lbs pressure (121°C) for 15 minutes. Allow the medium to set in sloped form with a butt about 1inch long.

Appendix-III: Indicators and Reagents

Andrade's Indicator

Acid Fucsin (0.5% aqueous solution)	500 ml
N-NaOH Solution	10 ml

(Add NaOH solution until solution becomes transparent; allow standing for 24 hours and filter it)

Acid- Alcohol

(For Ziehl Nielsen Stain)

HCL	3 ml
95% Ethyl Alcohol	100 ml

Chromic Acid Cleaning Solution

Potassium dichromate	80 gm.
Distilled water	300 ml
Conc. H_2SO_4	460 ml

Dissolve potassium dichromate in water and add acid slowly and carefully. Chromic Acid cleaning solution can be used repeatedly until it begins to turn green, when it should be discarded. Great care should be taken when preparing and handling this cleaning solution as it is extremely corrosive. Use protective clothing.

Kovac's Reagent

(For indole test)

Ingredients	
p-dimethylaminobenzaldehyde	10 gm.
Isoamyl Alcohol	150 ml
Concentrated Hydrochloric Acid	50 ml

Dissolve 10 gm. of p-dimethyl aminobenzaldehyde in 150 ml of isoamyl alcohol and then slowly adding 50 ml of concentrated hydrochloric acid.

Andrade Peptone Water

Ingredients	**g/l**
Peptic digest of animal tissue	10.000
Sodium chloride	5.000
Andrade indicator	0.100
Final pH (at 25°C) 7.5±0.2	

Directions

Suspend above ingredients in 1000 ml distilled water. Heat if necessary to dissolve the media ingredients completely. Adjust the pH and sterilize by autoclaving at 10lbs pressure (115°C) for 20 min. Cool to room temperature and aseptically add sterile stock solution of carbohydrate to a final concentration of 1.0% (w/v). Distribute in sterile test tubes.

Alkaline Peptone Water

Ingredients	**g/l**
Peptic digest of animal tissue	10.0
Sodium chloride	5.0
Final pH (at 25°C) 8.2 ± 0.2	

Directions

Suspend above ingredients in1000 ml distilled water. Heat if necessary to dissolve the medium completely. Adjust the pH and sterilize by autoclaving at 15lbs pressure (121°C) for 15 minutes.

Appendix-IV:

Table 1: Most Probable Number (MPN) of Organisms Per 100 ml of Sample and Confidence Limits Using 1 Tube of 50 ml, 5 Tubes of 10 ml and 5 Tubes of 1 ml

Number of Positive Tubes			**Most probable number (MPN)**	**Limits within which MPN per 100 ml can lie**	
50 ml tubes	**10 ml tubes**	**1 ml tubes**	**per 100 ml**	**Lower limit**	**Upper limit**
(1)	(2)	(3)	(4)	(5)	(6)
0	0	1	1	<0.5	4
0	0	2	2	<0.5	6
0	1	0	1	<0.5	4
0	1	1	2	<0.5	6
0	1	2	3	<0.5	8
0	2	0	2	<0.5	6
0	2	1	3	<0.5	8
0	2	2	4	<0.5	11
0	3	0	3	<0.5	8
0	3	1	5	<0.5	13
0	4	0	5	<0.5	13
1	0	0	1	<0.5	4
1	0	1	3	<0.5	8
1	0	2	4	<0.5	11
1	0	3	6	<0.5	15
1	1	0	3	<0.5	8
1	1	1	5	<0.5	13
1	1	2	7	1	17
1	1	3	9	2	21
1	2	0	5	<0.5	13
1	2	1	7	1	17
1	2	2	10	3	23
1	2	3	12	3	28
1	3	0	8	2	19
1	3	1	11	3	26
1	3	2	14	4	34
1	3	3	18	5	53

1	3	4	21	6	66
1	4	0	13	4	31
1	4	1	17	5	47
1	4	2	22	7	69
1	4	3	28	8	85
1	4	4	35	12	101
1	4	5	43	15	117
1	5	0	24	8	75
1	5	1	35	12	101
1	5	2	54	18	138
1	5	3	92	27	217
1	5	4	161	39	450

Table 2: Most Probable Number (MPN) of Organisms Present Per 100 ml of Sample and Confidance Limits Using 5 Tubes of 10 ml, 5 Tubes of 1 ml and 5 Tubes of 0.1 ml

Number of Positive Tubes			**Most probable number (MPN)**	**Limits within which MPN per 100 ml can lie**	
10 ml tubes	**1 ml tubes**	**0.1ml tubes**	**per 100 ml**	**Lower limit**	**Upper limit**
(1)	**(2)**	**(3)**	**(4)**	**(5)**	**(6)**
0	0	1	2	<0.5	7
0	0	2	4	<0.5	11
0	1	0	2	<0.5	7
0	1	1	4	<0.5	11
0	1	2	6	<0.5	15
0	2	0	4	<0.5	11
0	2	1	6	<0.5	15
0	3	0	6	<0.5	15
1	0	0	2	<0.5	7
1	0	1	4	<0.5	11
1	0	2	6	<0.5	15
1	0	3	8	1	19
1	1	0	4	<0.5	11
1	1	1	6	<0.5	15
1	1	2	8	1	19
1	2	0	6	<0.5	15

1	2	1	8	1	19
1	2	2	10	2	23
1	3	0	8	1	19
1	3	1	10	2	23
1	4	0	11	2	25
2	0	0	5	<0.5	13
2	0	1	7	1	17
2	0	2	9	2	21
2	0	3	12	3	28
2	1	0	7	1	17
2	1	1	9	2	21
2	1	2	12	3	28
2	2	0	9	2	21
2	2	1	12	3	28
2	2	2	14	4	34
2	3	0	12	3	28
2	3	1	14	4	34
2	4	0	15	4	37
3	0	0	8	1	19
3	0	1	11	2	25
3	0	2	13	3	31
3	1	0	11	2	25
3	1	1	14	4	34
3	1	2	17	5	46
3	1	3	20	6	60
3	2	0	14	4	34
3	2	1	17	5	46
3	2	2	20	6	60
3	3	0	17	5	46
3	3	1	21	7	63
3	4	0	21	7	63
3	4	1	24	8	72
3	5	0	25	8	75
4	0	0	13	3	31
4	0	1	17	5	46
4	0	2	21	7	63

4	0	2	25	8	75
4	1	0	17	5	46
4	1	1	21	7	63
4	1	2	26	9	78
4	2	0	22	7	67
4	2	1	26	9	78
4	2	2	32	11	91
4	3	0	27	9	80
4	3	1	33	11	93
4	3	2	39	13	106
4	4	0	34	12	96
4	4	1	40	14	108
4	5	0	41	14	110
4	5	1	48	16	124
5	0	0	23	7	70
5	0	1	31	11	89
5	0	2	43	15	114
5	0	3	58	19	144
5	0	4	76	24	180
5	1	0	33	11	93
5	1	1	46	16	120
5	1	2	63	21	154
5	1	3	84	26	197
5	2	0	49	17	126
5	2	1	70	23	168
5	2	2	94	28	219
5	2	3	120	33	281
5	2	4	148	38	366
5	2	5	177	44	515
5	3	0	79	25	187
5	3	1	109	31	253
5	3	2	141	37	343
5	3	3	175	44	503
5	3	4	212	53	669
5	3	5	253	77	788
5	4	0	130	35	302

5	4	1	172	43	486
5	4	2	221	57	698
5	4	3	278	90	849
5	4	4	345	117	999
5	4	5	426	145	1161
5	5	0	240	68	754
5	5	1	343	118	1005
5	5	2	542	180	1405

Table 3: Most Probable Number (MPN) of Organisms Present Per 100 ml of Sample and Confidance Limit Using 5 Tubes of 10 ml, 5 Tubes of 1 ml and 5 Tubes of 0.1 ml

Combination of positives	**MPN Index/**	**95% confidence limit**		**Combination of positives**	**MPN Index/**	**95% confidence limit**	
	100 ml	**Lower**	**Upper**		**100 ml**	**Lower**	**Upper**
0-0-0	<2	-	-	4-2-0	22	9.0	56
0-0-1	2	1.0	10	4-2-1	26	12	65
0-1-0	2	1.0	10	4-3-0	27	12	67
0-2-0	2	1.0	13	4-3-1	33	15	77
				4-4-0	34	16	80
				5-0-0	23	9.0	86
1-0-0	2	1.0	11	5-0-1	30	10	110
1-0-1	4	1.0	15	5-0-2	40	20	140
1-1-0	4	1.0	15	5-1-0	30	10	120
1-1-1	6	2.0	18	5-1-1	50	20	150
1-2-0	6	2.0	18	5-1-2	60	30	180
2-0-0	4	1.0	17	5-2-0	50	20	170
2-0-1	7	2.0	20	5-2-1	70	30	210
2-1-0	7	2.0	21	5-2-2	90	40	250
2-1-1	9	3.0	24	5-3-0	80	30	250
2-2-0	9	3.0	25	5-3-1	11	40	300
2-3-0	12	5.0	29	5-3-2	140	60	360
3-0-0	8	3.0	24	5-3-3	170	80	410
3-0-1	11	4.0	29	5-4-0	130	50	390
3-1-0	11	4.0	29	5-4-1	170	70	480
3-1-1	14	6.0	35	5-4-2	220	100	580

3-2-0	14	6.0	35	5-4-3	280	120	690
3-2-1	17	7.0	40	5-4-4	350	160	820
				5-5-0	240	100	940
4-0-0	13	5.70	38	5-5-1	300	100	1300
4-0-1	17	7.0	45	5-5-2	500	200	2000
4-1-0	17	7.0	46	5-5-3	900	300	2900
4-1-1	21	9.0	55	5-5-4	1600	600	5300
4-1-2	26	12.0	63	5-5-5	1600	-	-

Table 4: Most Probable Number (MPN) of Organisms Present Per 100 ml of Sample and Confidence Limit Using 1 Tubes of 50 ml and 5 Tubes of 10 ml

Number of positive tubes		**Most probable number (MPN)**	**Limits within which MPN per 100 ml can lie**	
50 ml tubes	**10 ml tubes**	**per 100 ml**	**Lower limit**	**Upper limit**
(1)	**(2)**	**(3)**	**(4)**	**(5)**
0	1	1	<0.5	4
0	2	2	<0.5	6
0	3	4	<0.5	11
0	4	5	1	13
1	0	2	<0.5	6
1	1	3	<0.5	9
1	2	6	1	15
1	3	9	2	21
1	4	16	4	40

Bibliography

Aneja, K. R. (2010). Experiments in Microbiology, Plant Pathology and Biotechnology. New Age Publishers, New Delhi, India

APHA (1992). Standard Methods for the Examination of Dairy Products. American Public Health Assoication, Washington, D.C.

Atlas, R. M. & Parks, L. C. (1997). Handbook of Microbiological Media. International Publishers, New Delhi. 2nd ed. CRC Press, Boca Raton,

Benson, H., J. (1990). Microbiological Applications. A laboratory manual in general microbiology. 5th Ed. C. brown Publishers: USA.

Enzymology, Practical Manual BIOC231, Kingdom of Saudi Arabia, King Abdulaziz University, Girls Collage of Science, Biochemistry Department.

FSSAI (2023). Manual of Methods of Analysis- Microbiological Examination of Food and Water. Food Safety Standards Authority of India, New Delhi.

Marshall, R. T. (1992). Standard Methods for the Examination of Dairy Products. 16th Ed. APHA, Washington.

Meena, K. K., Goel, D. & Mali, A. (2019). Practical Manual On: Food & Industrial Microbiology.

Meena, K. K., Mudgal, V. D. & Kumar, A. (2019). Introductory Microbiology (A Practical Book). Agrotech Publishing Academy, Udaipur. ISBN: 978-81-8321-518-3

Prajapati, J. B., Reddy, I. S. & Sreeja, V. (2012). Starter Culture & Fermented Milk Products. ICAR- e-course.

Colour Plates

Chapter 4

Parts of the Light Microscope

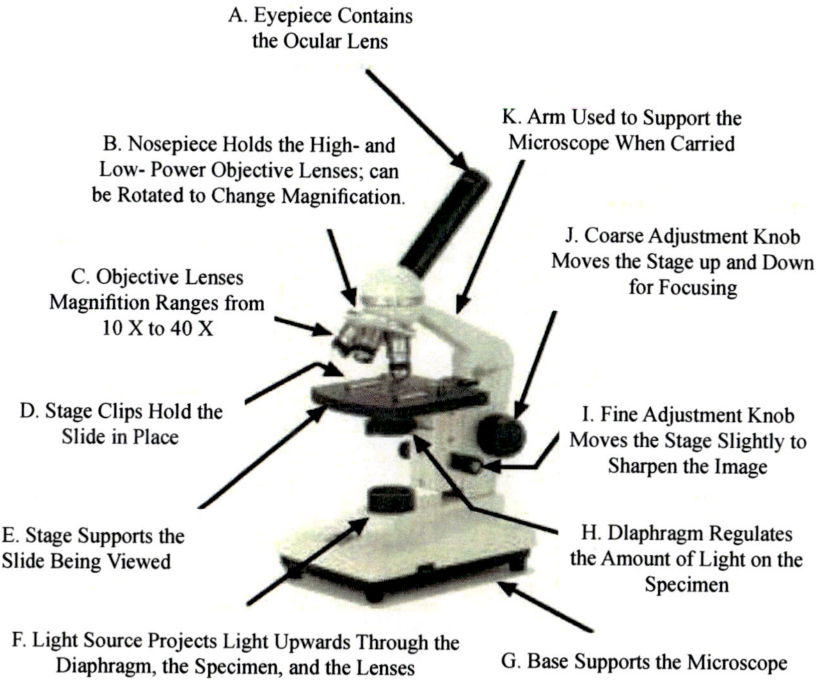

Fig.: Parts of Light Microscope

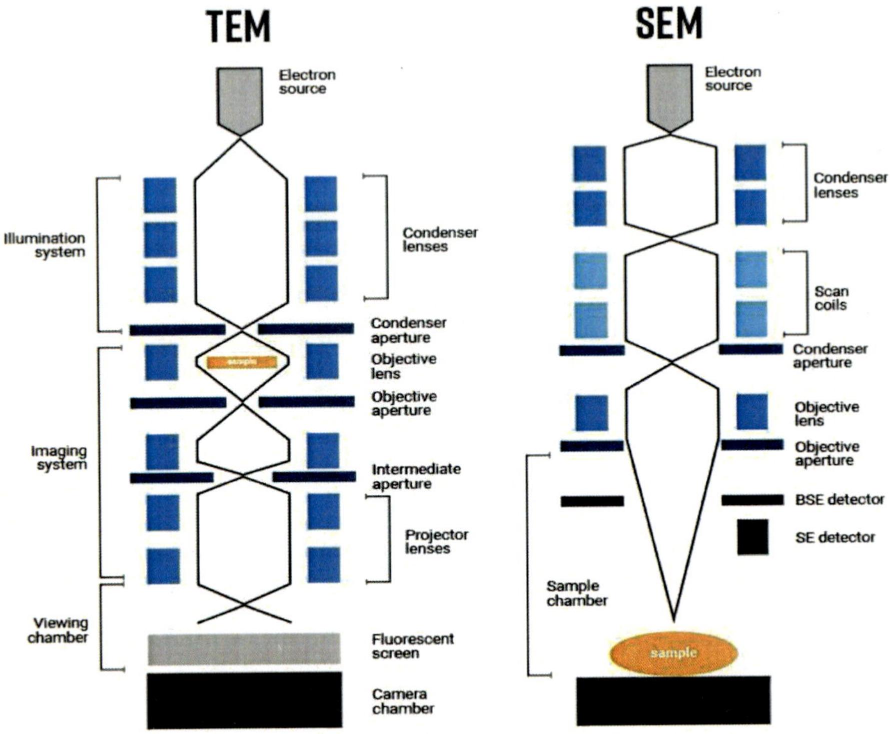

Fig. : Schematic diagram of TEM vs SEM (Courtesy: https://www.nanoscience.com)

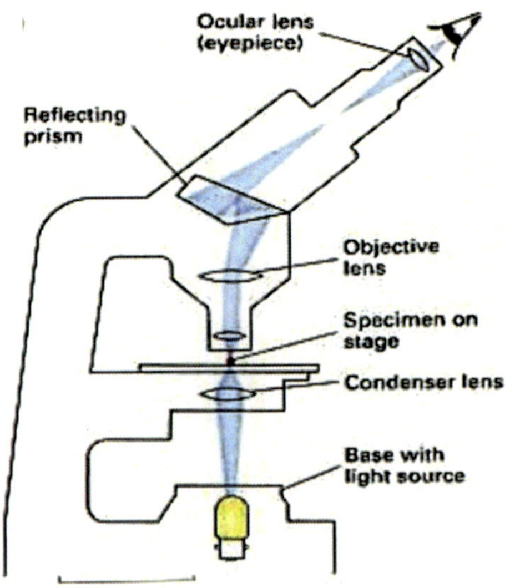

Fig. : Bright Field Microscope

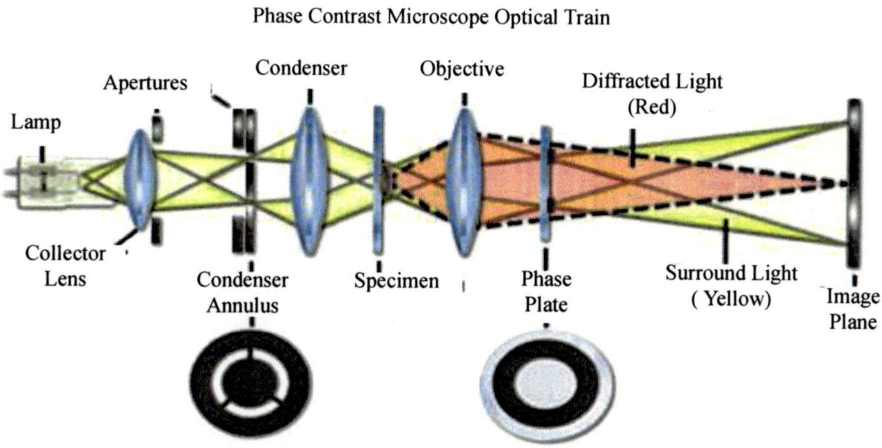

Fig. : Light Path Phase Contrast Microscope

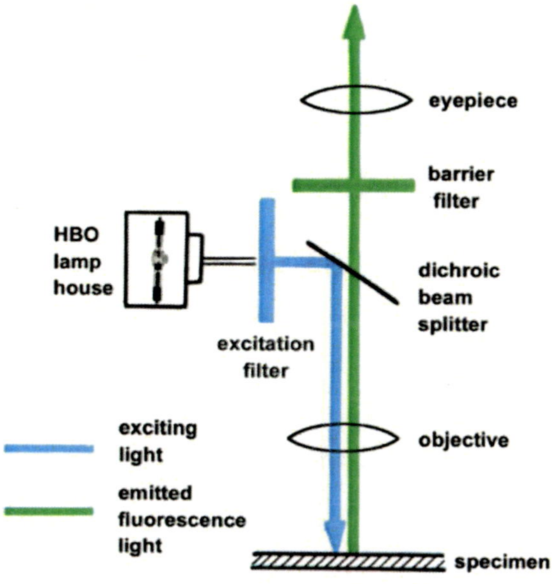

Fig. : Light Path in Fluorescence Microscope

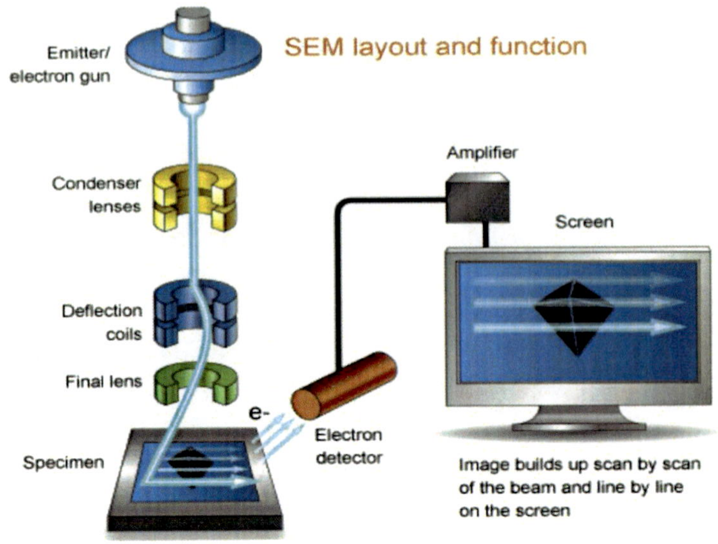

Fig. : SEM Layout

Chapter 6

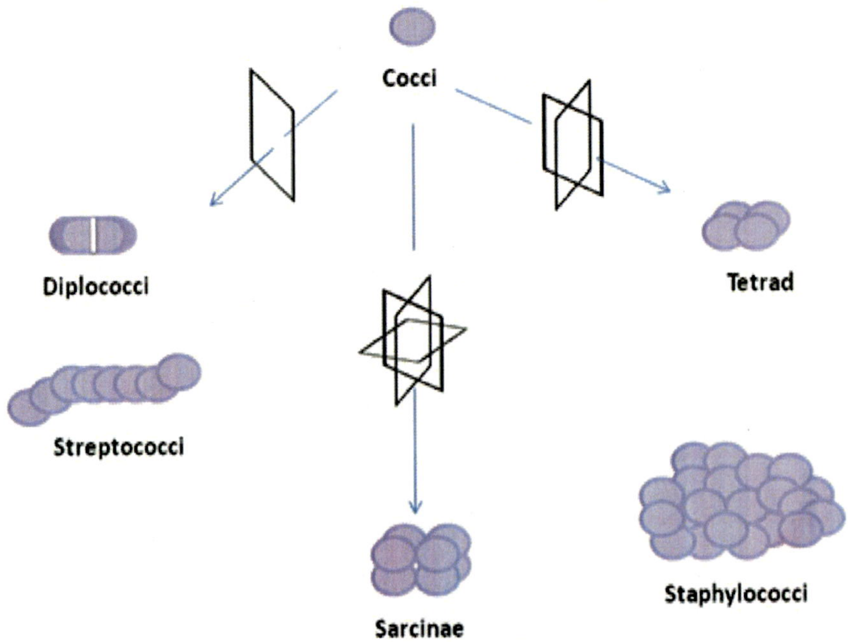

Fig. : Arrangement of Cocci

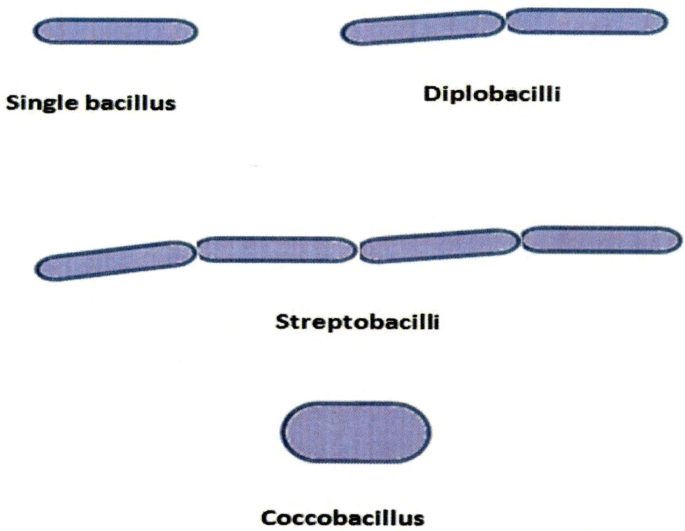

Fig. : Arrangement of Bacilli

Chapter 8

Gram (+) and Gram (-) Cell Walls

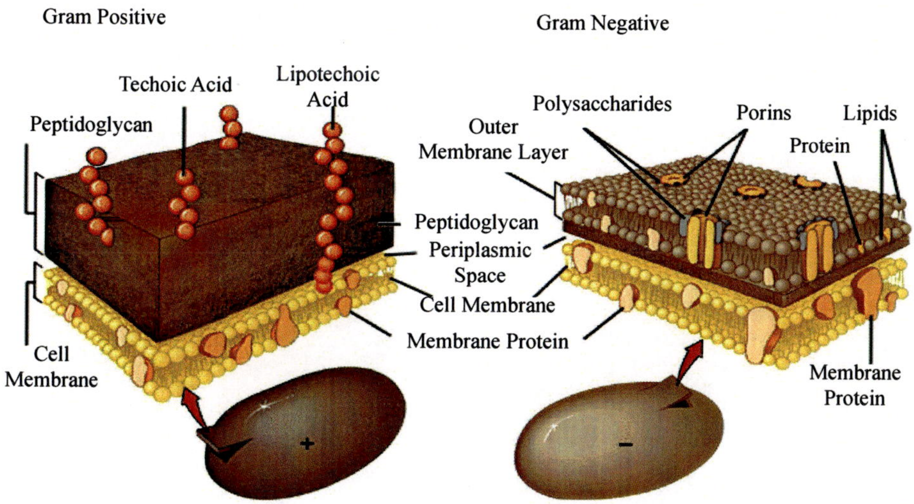

Fig. : Gram Positive and Gram Negative Cell Walls

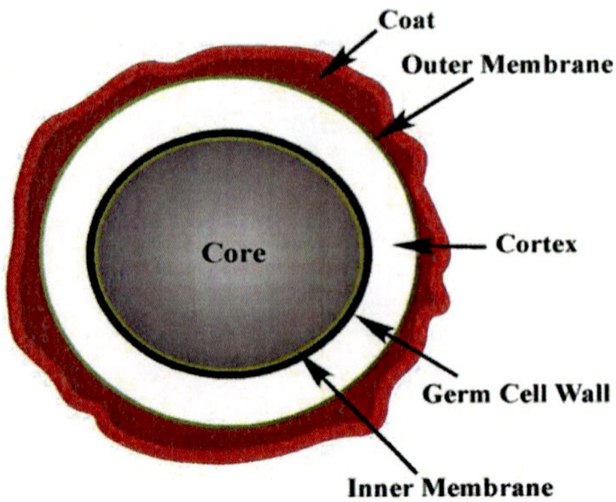

Fig. : Structure of Spore

Chapter 13

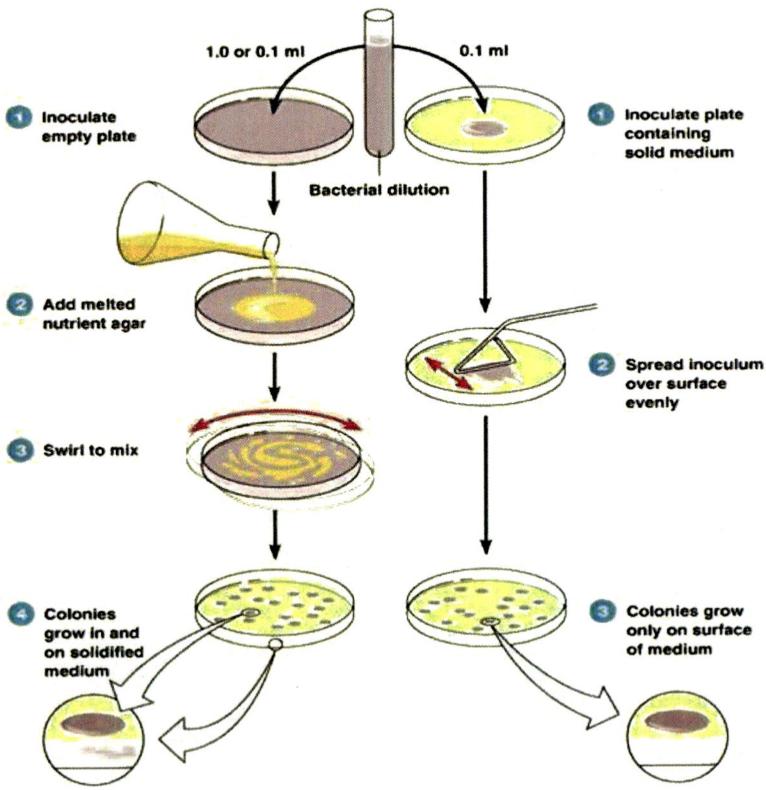

Fig. : Spread Plate Technique (Courtesy: www.canava.com)

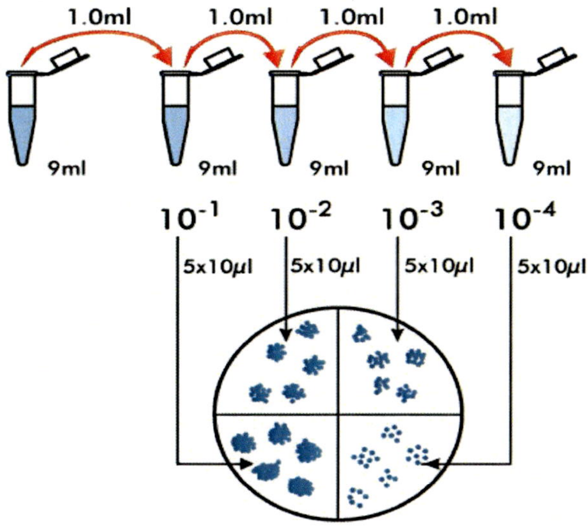

Fig. : Drop Plate Technique (Courtesy: www.canava.com)

Chapter 15

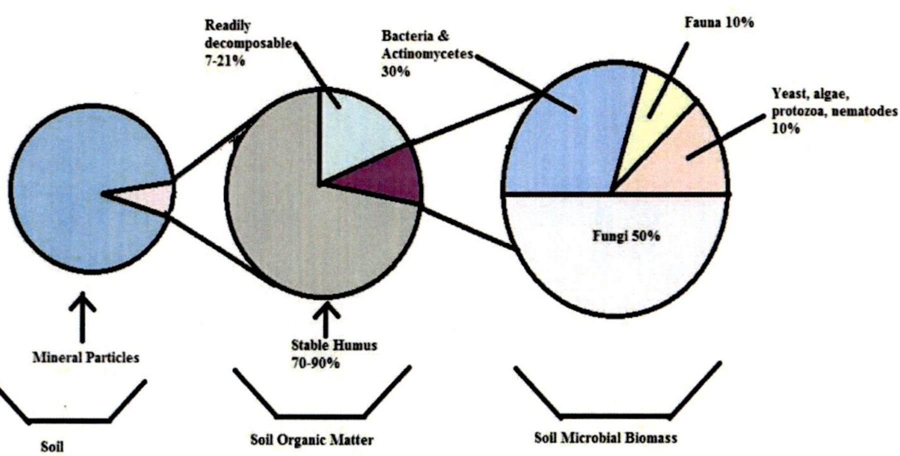

Fig. Major components of soil

Scientific Index